STRONG

STRONG

ZANNA VAN DIJK

HEADLINE

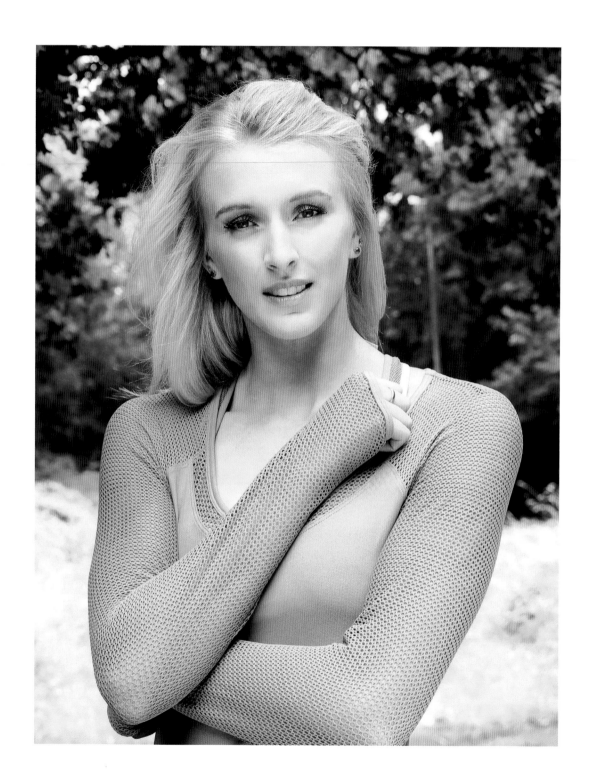

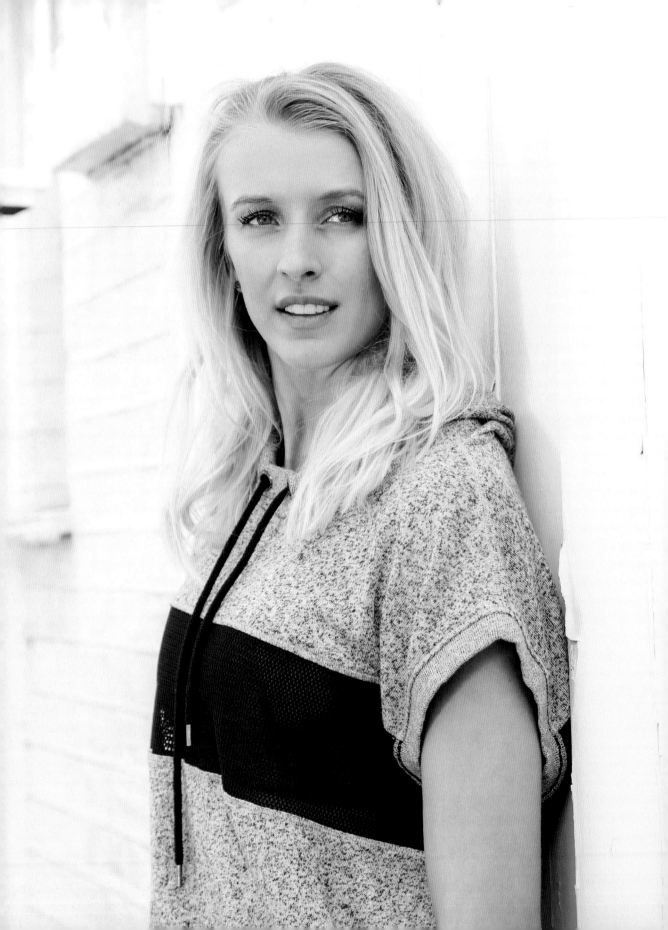

Every single day we are bombarded with information about the latest diet craze or weight loss quick-fix – from exercising while wrapped in cling film (yes, really!) through to juice cleanses, detox teas and everything in between.

Quite frankly it can be overwhelming and confusing, and can lead you down a road of yo-yo dieting, losing and regaining weight, and never truly finding a lifestyle which you can stick to.

What if I told you that you don't need to follow these radical approaches to feel energised, lose weight, get fitter and achieve lasting results?

It's all about finding *balance.*

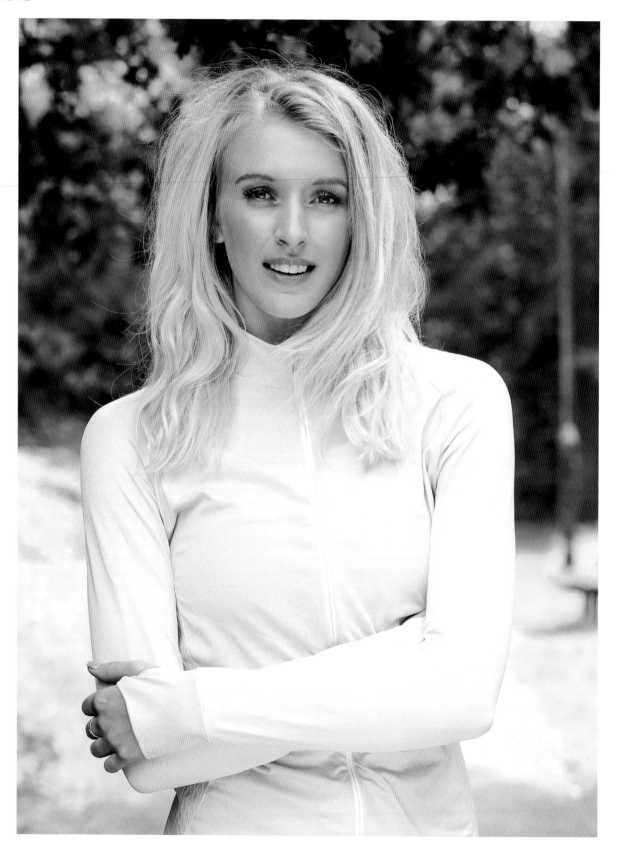

MY JOURNEY

When I was at school, staying healthy certainly wasn't high on my priority list. I would do anything to avoid exercise. I wrote fake sick notes for P.E. on a regular basis and struggled to run for the bus. I would eat sugary cereal for breakfast, have pasta and brownies for lunch, and snack on sausage rolls. I saw working out as a chore and eating healthily as uncool, and this attitude stuck with me into early adulthood.

When I was at university I gained the 'freshers' 15 (pounds)' and as a result I made it my mission to lose weight through any method possible. I tried every diet out there. I'm talking low carb, high carb, paleo, the cabbage soup diet... you name it, I did it. I ended up slimmer but tired, fed up and frustrated. I wasn't enjoying my food and I was about as active as a sloth. It was at this point that I decided to prioritise my health. I was tired of feeling tired and I wanted to learn how to nourish my body and get fit and strong the right way.

Being the nerd that I am, I dived head first into a mountain of books on the topic of health and kept up with the latest research in the area. I soon realised that the fad diets I had been following were a load of nonsense and that there is so much more to training than plodding along on a treadmill. I educated myself about how to fuel my body appropriately, the importance of macronutrients, the value of strength training and so much more. I started to implement this knowledge on myself and the results came thick and fast. I became energised, my concentration improved and my skin glowed. I started to enjoy my training, I developed muscle tone and I became stronger than I ever thought I could be. Instead of seeing food as the enemy, I saw it as something to be enjoyed. I started using it as fuel to nourish my body. Instead of seeing exercise as a chore, I saw it as a way to look after myself and a gateway to thrive both physically and mentally.

Health and fitness soon went from being a hobby to a passion, and after I left university I studied to become a personal trainer. Now I make it my mission to educate others about having a balanced approach to fitness and nutrition so that they don't make the mistakes I did. I ensure that everyone I work with looks beyond their appearance and considers how they feel. I am constantly learning through continued professional development, reading books, attending workshops and listening to hours of podcasts. I want to challenge you to change your beliefs and change your life. I want **you** to feel awesome, energised and empowered. I strongly believe that life is for living, food is for eating and exercise is to be enjoyed. Gone are the days of restrictive diets and hours of exercise. Say hello to an achievable, realistic and enjoyable approach to looking after your body, losing weight and thriving every single day. Say hello to **balance**.

THE BOOK

How many times have you been told, 'It's not a diet, it's a lifestyle'? What does that even mean? How do you actually live this elusive *lifestyle* everyone talks about? That is what this book is here to tell you.

Strong avoids strict diet plans, busts fitness myths and tells you what you **actually** need to know so that you can enjoy your journey to becoming healthier. It is not an unsustainable short-term fix that leaves you tired, weak and deprived. It isn't a cleanse and it certainly isn't a detox. It is a detailed guide crammed full of information which you can use to educate yourself about how to fuel your body, train hard and achieve a healthy lifestyle for the long term. It guides you through how to make small healthy choices which fit into **your** life, as it is these daily decisions that ultimately determine your health, happiness and results.

A balanced approach emphasises both body and mind. Not only do you need to learn how to cook delicious food and push yourself in the gym but you also need to make sure you have the mindset to match. As a result, not only will we discuss slotting fitness into your life and reducing stress but we will also make sure you maintain a positive relationship with food and with your body along the way. By the time you finish reading this book, you'll be a balanced badass with so much knowledge that it'll be coming out of your ears!

Now I don't want to get ahead of myself here… but this book has the potential to change your life. Yep, bold statement. However, if you just read it and then pop it on a shelf never to be touched again, that probably won't happen. Instead, I encourage you to really engage with the information I present to you, absorb it and question it. Grab a pen, write in the margins, fold down corners, make notes and be inquisitive. Get nerdy, ask questions and look further into areas that interest you. I will give you as many tools and tips as I can but don't stop there. This book is a starting point on what I hope will be a continuing journey for you as a reader.

Now, it's over to you. The power is in your hands to take control of your body, mind, health and life and to implement the changes you need to achieve long-lasting results. I hope that this book inspires you to cook delicious meals, train like a badass, achieve a balanced lifestyle and feel pretty damn amazing along the way.

Zanna xx

Disclaimer: It's always a good idea to check with your doctor before making significant changes to your lifestyle, especially if you haven't exercised for a while or have a medical condition. Don't push yourself on the exercise front unless you know it's safe to do so.

This book is for you if...

You have lost weight and regained it in the past.

You're fed up with yo-yo dieting and nonsense quick-fixes.

You're overwhelmed by the mixed messages in the fitness industry.

You're bored by bland salads and the same old smoothies.

You're busy, stressed and short on time.

You struggle to get motivated to be healthy.

You want to get stronger in both body and mind.

You're tired and your skin is breaking out.

You want to make lasting healthy changes to your lifestyle.

You want to find a balanced approach which you can **enjoy**!

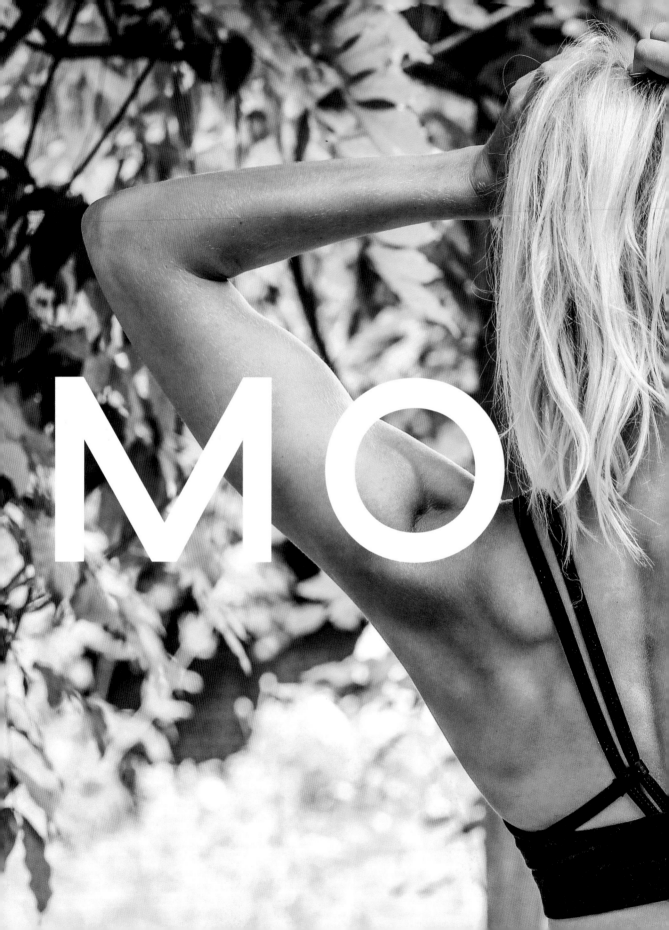

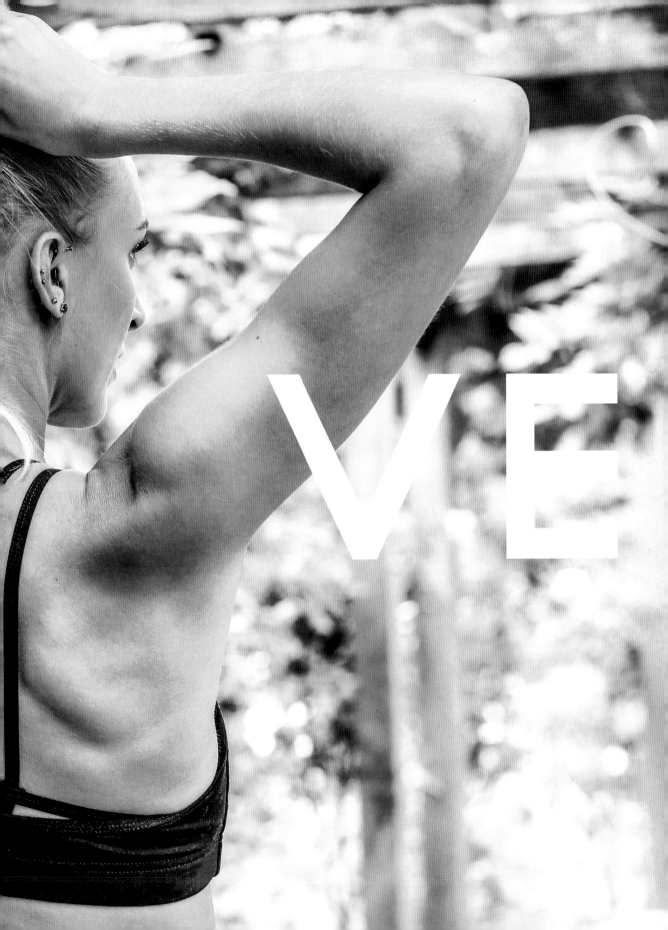

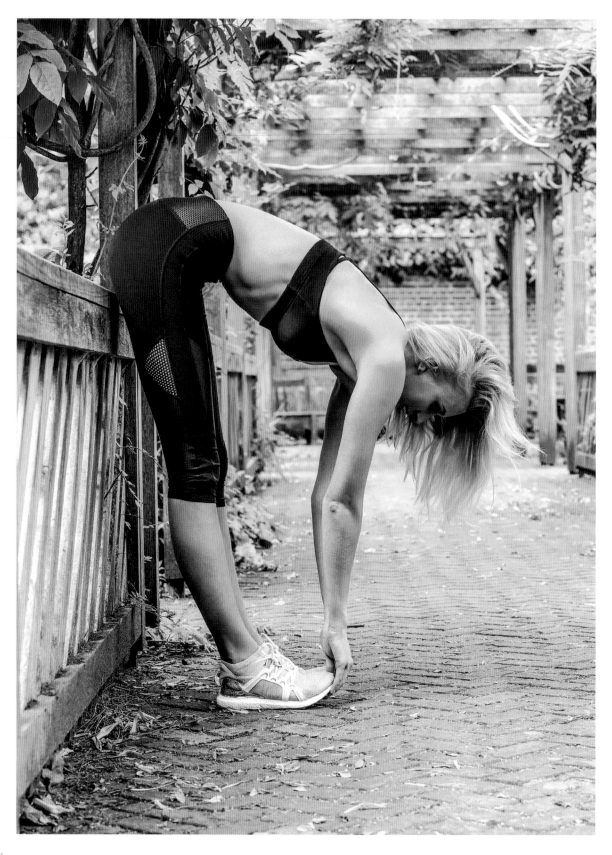

MOVE

Newsflash: exercise is essential! Not just because it makes you look and feel awesome, but because it vastly improves your health both physically and mentally. Along with good nutrition, moving your body is the best way to take care of yourself and to invest in your future. In reality, it is in our nature to be active. Your body wants to be fit and strong. It wants to be fast and powerful. It is just that in our modern-day lives, in which we spend the vast majority of our time sitting down in cars, at desks and on sofas, we aren't living up to our potential.

Exercise is often seen as a chore – something to be suffered through to cancel out that slice of cake we ate last night. It doesn't have to be this way. I strongly believe that exercise can be enjoyable, and enjoyment leads to sustainability. There are so many ways you can move now, from Pilates and weight training through to bouncing on mini-trampolines and dancing in unitards. There is quite literally something for everyone! However, that's not to say that from the get-go you're going to fall in love with working out. Honestly, it will be a challenge at first. You will feel uncomfortable and you will want to stop. Your body will be thinking 'what the hell are you doing to me?' and that little voice in your head will say 'why don't you just go home and make brownies instead?'.

You need to go into a workout accepting that it will be a challenge. Exercising **should** push you out of your comfort zone, because that's when you get the best results! I pinky promise that once you get a series of good workouts under your belt, you will be feeling like an absolute goddess and will want to go back for more. There is nothing more satisfying than that post-workout feeling! Not only will you feel fitter, stronger and healthier but your skin will glow, you'll let off some steam, you'll sleep better and you'll feel more energised. Plus, the more you move, the more you can eat... it's a no-brainer really!

MY TOP FITNESS PRINCIPLES

SUSTAINABILITY IS KEY

There is no quick fix. You can't just train for 12 weeks and then call it a day. Becoming fitter is an ongoing process with no end date, so you need to find something you can stick to.

CHALLENGE YOURSELF

If you breeze through a workout and don't feel like you worked very hard, you probably didn't, and the results will reflect that. You need to push your body well and truly out of your comfort zone to make significant changes to your fitness levels and your physique.

GET STRONG

The benefits of lifting weights are endless. I recommend that every person does some form of resistance training to not only feel like a badass but also sculpt a good ass!

LESS IS MORE

Most of us haven't got time to spend hours in the gym. Although your workouts need to be hard, they don't need to be long. Intensity is more important than duration. Quality over quantity.

GET MOVING

Cardio can be hardio, but again the benefits are huge. Whether you go for a long walk in the park or do some high-intensity hill sprints, get a sweat on to improve your physical and psychological health.

RECOVERY IS ESSENTIAL

There is so much more to being fit than just working out. You need to support your recovery with sleep, stretching and stress reduction. Oh and don't forget those vital rest days!

DON'T SWEAT THE SMALL STUFF

People often get hung up on tiny details such as what time of day they train. These don't matter in the grand scheme of things. What is really important is that you fit exercising into **your** life and that you do it **consistently**.

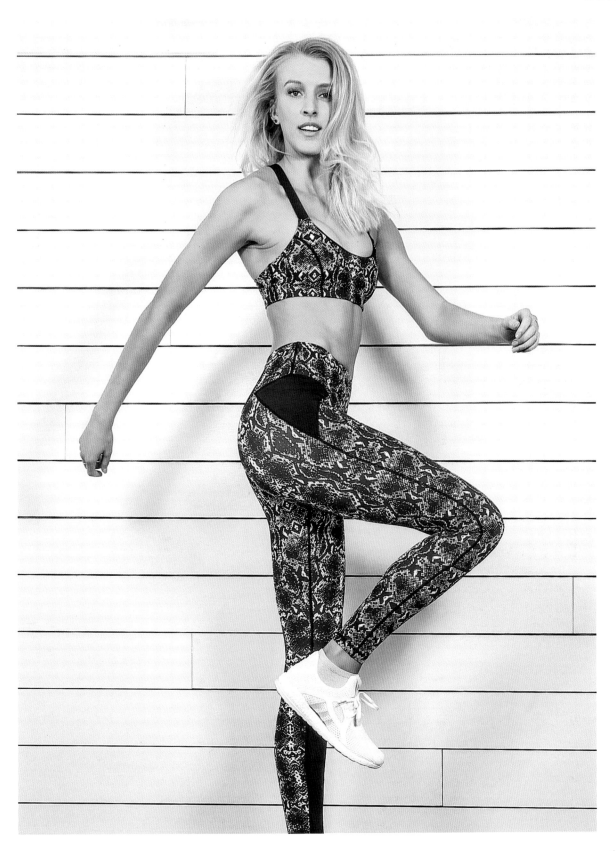

"Your only limit is you."

RESISTANCE TRAINING

THE BENEFITS OF LIFTING

Want to know the secret to feeling strong, powerful and fierce? Lifting weights. Lifting weights makes you feel like a badass by building lean muscle tissue, but don't be put off by those words. I don't mean 'building' in the sense of growing huge biceps to flex on magazine covers. I mean building a body that is strong, fit, toned and capable of carrying you through life. Through resistance training you can strengthen not only your muscles but also your bones. Resistance training improves bone density and reduces your chances of developing osteoporosis, something post-menopausal women are particularly at risk of.

The benefits don't stop there though. Lifting weights supports any other form of training – such as running, cycling or swimming – by developing muscular strength. Furthermore, by building up lean muscle, you can quite literally sculpt your body and build curves in all the right places. Always wanted a peachy bum or defined arms? There's a weighted workout for that. By developing muscle mass you also become a fat-burning machine. Your body has to burn more calories to maintain a kilo of muscle than it does to maintain a kilo of fat. The more you build, the more you burn. Say hello to a faster metabolism and improved energy levels!

Perhaps the most valuable benefit of resistance training though, and the main reason why I love it so much, is becoming stronger both mentally and physically. Lifting weights enables you to function better in everyday life. You can open jars without asking for help (pass me the peanut butter...). You can carry your shopping, lift your children and move furniture with ease. And, by developing yourself physically, you become healthier mentally. You become more confident, independent and empowered. You feel happier from the endorphins and less stressed from letting off steam. Basically, you will feel and look pretty damn amazing, so don't be afraid to pick up some heavy weights!

Busting myths: So many girls think that lifting weights will make them become big and bulky. That is a load of bull. If it was that easy do you think that men would spend so many hours in the gym zealously trying to grow their biceps? Building muscle is a steady process and takes time, especially for us ladies. You won't end up looking like The Hulk — I promise!

BRAVING THE 'TESTOSTER-ZONE'

So, you've never stepped foot in the weights section of the gym and, quite frankly, you're bricking it. Thoughts are racing through your head: 'What will everyone think? Won't I stand out like a sore thumb? What if I make a fool out of myself?' Trust me, I've been there and I've felt that. For the first few months that I lifted weights I never stepped into the weights room. I would sneak off to a quiet corner of the gym with my dumbbells and do my thing in peace. It was only once I felt confident with lifting that I actually dared to enter what I now fondly call the testoster-zone. It was then that I realised that there is nothing to fear and, in fact, I wished I had gone in there in the first place! Here's why:

• By going into the weights section, you will have access to all the equipment you could ever need, from barbells and dumbbells to cable machines and the leg press. This means more tools available to sculpt your body.

• Everyone in the gym, whether they're doing cardio or resistance training, is there to better themselves. They are not there to judge other people, and, if they are, do you really care what they think? (Spoiler: don't!)

• Other gym-goers and the gym staff are often more than willing to help and will not judge you for asking for assistance. Everyone was once a beginner, and it is better to ask for advice than to do an exercise with poor form or to use a machine incorrectly.

• Most of the people in the weights room are too focused on themselves and their own programme to even bat an eyelid at what anyone else is doing. If someone does notice you, they're not going to be thinking negatively. They are most likely thinking how much they respect you for going in there!

So, fingers crossed I have convinced you to go and lift some weights. Now, here are my top tips for striding into that resistance room with confidence.

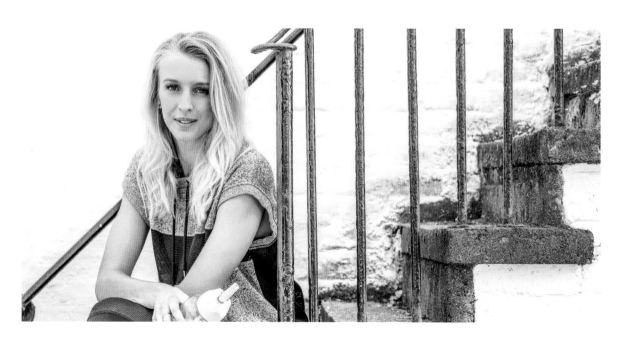

TOP TIPS FOR FEELING CONFIDENT IN THE GYM

MAKE A PLAN

Write down the exercises you want to do and how many sets and reps you want to achieve (or just take this book in with you). Make sure you're familiar with the exercises and know how to use correct form – YouTube is a great resource full of tutorials for even the most obscure moves.

ASK FOR AN INDUCTION

Most gyms give a free induction, which is your time to get a full interactive tour of the gym including the weights room. Take this opportunity to ask questions, request demonstrations and familiarise yourself with the facilities. Some gyms even offer a complimentary personal training session, so definitely take advantage of that and use the time wisely to learn good form on key exercises.

WEAR HEADPHONES

Make yourself a banging playlist packed full of your favourite tunes. Plug it in before you enter the weights room and let the music make you feel like a badass who doesn't care what anyone thinks!

BUDDY UP

Grab a friend and drag them to the gym with you – the weights room is so much easier to enter when you have a partner in crime. You can experiment with the equipment together and spur each other on through an awesome workout.

GET KITTED OUT

Wear a workout outfit which is both comfortable and flattering. Nothing kills your sassy vibe more than leggings which slip down when you squat!

TIME IT RIGHT

To ease yourself into it, try entering the weights room at an off-peak time (that means not just before or just after work). It will be quieter, giving you free rein to explore everything it has to offer.

FOCUS ON YOURSELF

Try to zone out from everyone else in the gym and focus on what you're doing and why you're doing it. Concentrate on your form rather than on other gym-goers. After all, you're here for you and no one else.

FAKE IT TILL YOU MAKE IT

Strut into that weights room with a stride of pride and act like you've been in there loads of times. By simply telling yourself 'you've got this' and holding your head high, you will immediately feel more confident and powerful – and no one will have a clue that you're a newbie!

The first time you enter the weights room it will most likely be a bit daunting. However, it gets easier and easier every single time you go, until eventually it's second nature and you look back and question why you were ever nervous about it at all.

PSSSST! If you don't have a gym membership and going to a weights room simply isn't an option, I've got your back! This section contains a bunch of at-home weighted workouts too.

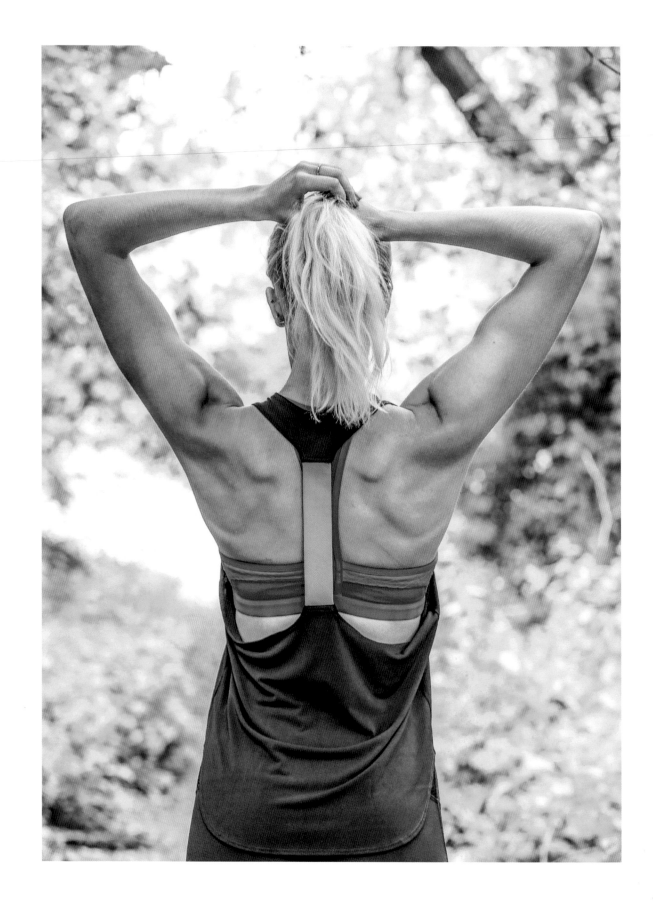

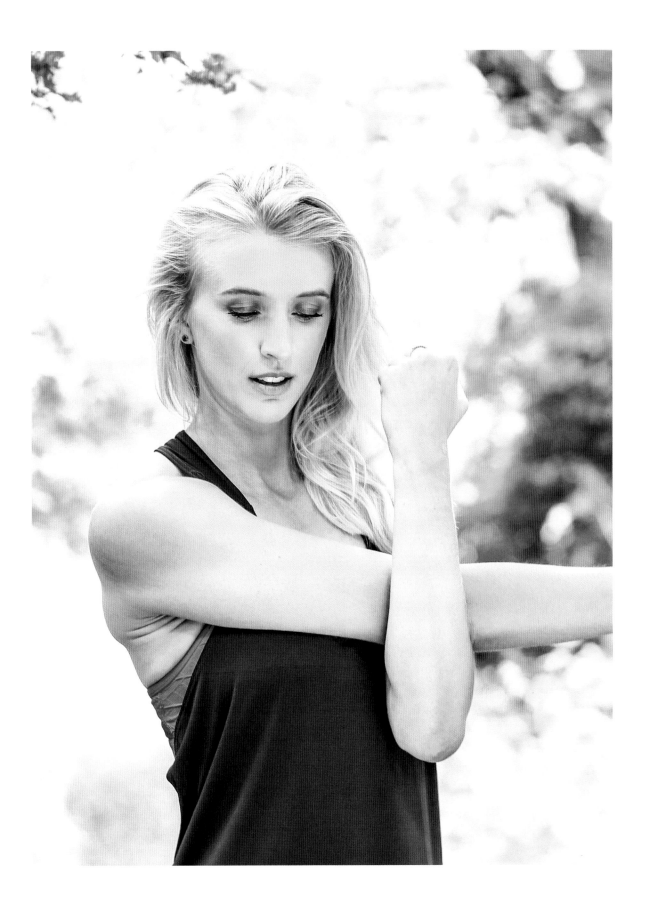

THE RESISTANCE WORKOUTS

So, this is how it's going to work. Now that I have convinced you to pick up some dumbbells, I am going to guide you through a series of weighted workouts. There are beginners' workouts which can be done at home, and advanced workouts which require equipment you can find at the gym. These are structured so that you can easily follow them, with sets and reps outlined for every move (more on that later!).

Alrighty, now let's get down to business. Weight training is a powerful and effective form of exercise which gives quick, visible and lasting results – so I understand why you want to get going right now! But, before you go squatting and lunging all over the gym, here are a few top tips for beginners that I think you should read.

TOP TIPS FOR LIFTING WEIGHTS

FOCUS ON FORM

Form means how you perform an exercise and it is **the** most important thing when it comes to weight training. Using correct form ensures that you will be targeting the right muscles and getting the most effective workout, and you will significantly reduce your risk of injury too. If you're ever unsure about how to perform an exercise, ask a trainer at your gym; they should be more than happy to help.

LIFT HEAVY

Gone are the days of light weights and high reps – if you want to torch fat and build lean muscle, you need to challenge yourself, ladies! I promise you, you are so much stronger than you ever imagined. Use weights which really push you out of your comfort zone, always maintaining that essential good form.

TRAIN YOUR WHOLE BODY

You might think it's a wise idea to train just a specific area you want to target, but in reality this can lead to muscular imbalances and injuries. Have you ever seen those guys in the gym who just train their chest and neglect their back, and as a result have poor posture? Instead, ensure you work every muscle group to lead to a balanced physique.

USE THE MIND–MUSCLE CONNECTION

Whenever you perform an exercise, really try to connect your mind with the muscle which you are using. Focus on it, engage it and contract it. Doing this actually helps to ensure you use the correct muscles and get the most from your workouts.

CHECK YOURSELF OUT

The weights room isn't full of mirrors just so that gym-goers can check out their abs; they're actually there for a reason! Don't be afraid to look at your reflection and check your form, to ensure you're doing the exercises correctly. It's not vain, it's safe.

BE CONSISTENT

Lifting weights has the power to completely transform your body – but only if you stick with it. Resistance training once a month isn't going to cut it. Try to do it once a week at first and then go from there. Once you see the results, you'll be hooked!

CHALLENGE YOURSELF

Get comfortable with being uncomfortable. Learn to push yourself further and harder in each workout. Every single session is a new opportunity to get stronger and fitter. You should always be trying to lift more weight or do more reps, provided you can do so with good form. Keep pushing yourself to avoid hitting a plateau.

DON'T RUSH

A key element of weight training is 'time under tension'. This basically means that the more time a muscle spends under resistance, the more strain it is put under and the better the results will be. If you rush through an exercise, you will most likely not be using your muscles to their full potential.

BREATHE

I often see people in the gym holding their breath while they lift weights, which is a huge no-no. Instead I recommend breathing out on the 'hard' part of a lift (which means when your body is going against the resistance) and breathing in on the 'easy' part.

ENGAGE YOUR CORE

This not only reduces the risk of lower back injury but also helps to develop, tone and tighten your tummy. I find that my abs can get an awesome workout just by being engaged during my weight-training routines. How can you do this effectively? The easiest way is to imagine someone is about to punch you in the stomach and brace your tummy ready for the impact. That feeling of tightness in your stomach is your core engaging.

BE AWARE OF YOUR LIMITATIONS

If you find certain exercises particularly challenging, have any injuries or have poor mobility in certain areas (such as your hips or shoulders), get it checked out. I also recommend consulting a physiotherapist, doctor or other health professional prior to starting any exercise programme. Take on board any recommendations they have and take it slow.

LOOK AFTER YOURSELF

Warm up, cool down, stretch and use a foam roller appropriately to release tension and reduce your risk of injury. Lifting weights causes micro-tears in your muscles and as they repair, they grow stronger. Take rest days to facilitate this. Listen to your body – if you're too sore or too tired, give yourself some time off. Just make sure that when you hit the gym again it's with some serious power and passion! If you **ever** feel any sharp pains, persistent niggles or recurring aches, stop what you're doing and go and see a physiotherapist or health professional. Injuries aren't fun.

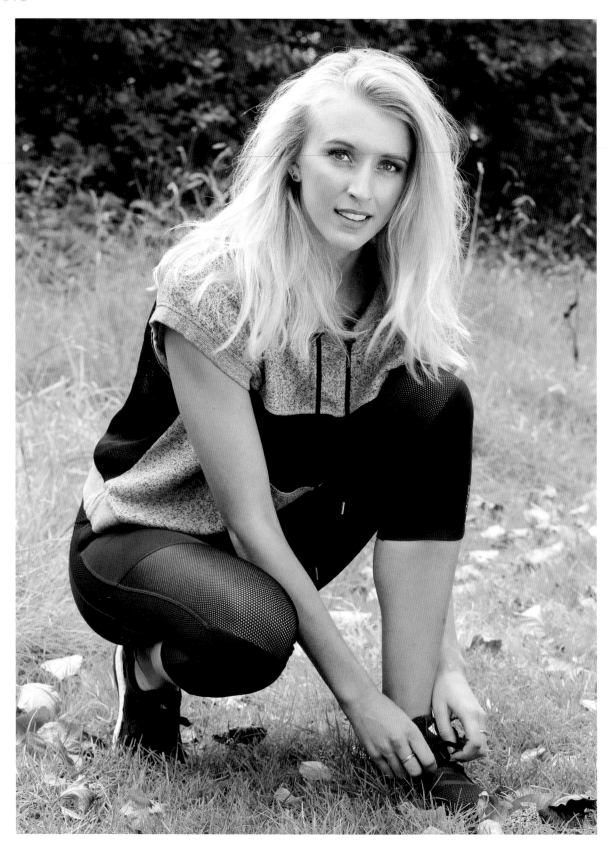

What are all these funky words?

REPETITION (REPS)
The number of times that you lift and lower a weight in one set of an exercise. For example, if you lift and lower a weight 10 times before setting the weight down, you have completed 10 'reps' in one set.

SET
A group of reps of an exercise after which you take a short rest period. For example, if you complete 10 reps, set the weight down, complete 10 more reps, set the weight down again, and repeat for a final 10 reps, you have completed three sets of the exercise.

REST
The pause between sets of an exercise, which allows muscles to recover partially before beginning the next set.

STRAIGHT SETS
Performing all sets of one exercise (including rest periods in between) before moving on to the next exercise.

SUPERSETS
Performing two exercises consecutively (back to back) without a break. You rest after you have completed both moves.

TRISETS
Performing three exercises consecutively (back to back) without a break. You rest after you have completed all three moves.

GIANT SETS
Performing four (or more) exercises consecutively (back to back) without a break. You rest after you have completed all four moves.

DROP SETS
A technique where you perform a set of an exercise and then immediately reduce the weight and perform another set of the same exercise using this lighter weight until you can't do any more reps.

COMPOUND EXERCISES
Compound exercises are multi-joint movements that work several muscles or muscle groups at one time. Examples are squats and deadlifts.

ISOLATION EXERCISES
Isolation exercises are movements that involve only one joint and a limited number of muscle groups. An example is a dumbbell bicep curl.

MUSCLE CONTRACTIONS
A *concentric* contraction causes muscles to shorten, thereby generating force. An example is the upwards phase of a bicep curl. *Eccentric* contractions cause muscles to elongate in response to a greater opposing force. An example is the lowering phase of a bicep curl. *Isometric* contractions generate force without changing a muscle's length. An example is holding a plank.

MY WARM-UP AND COOL-DOWN ROUTINES

THE WARM UP

Warming up is absolutely essential when weight training. You wouldn't just hop on a treadmill and start sprinting, and it's exactly the same with weighted workouts. You need to loosen up your joints, warm up your muscles and get your body moving before you start putting it under resistance. This increases blood flow to your muscles, helps to improve your range of motion so that you can perform exercises more effectively, and reduces the risk of injury. To warm up I recommend using dynamic stretches and movements which increase your body temperature and heart rate to prepare you for exercise. These also help to fire up your nervous system so it is ready to move some heavy weights. Here are some examples of my favourite moves.

Top tip: These warm-up and cool-down recommendations should be used when you're doing the bodyweight workouts too!

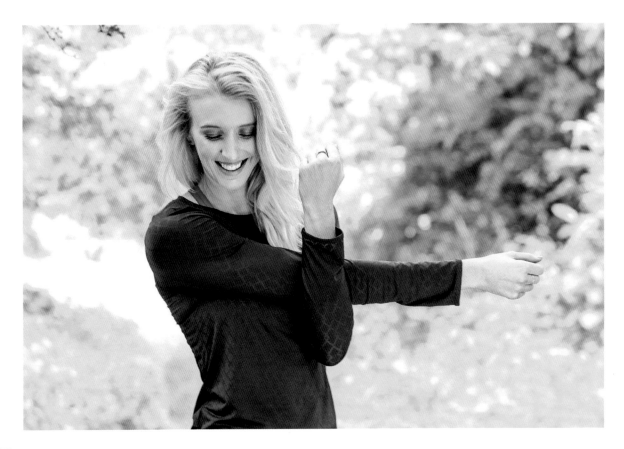

UPPER BODY

ARM CIRCLES

Stand in an upright position, bring your arms up so they are in line with your shoulders and then bend them. Start to move the arms in a circular motion forwards and backwards, warming up the shoulder joint. These can also be performed with straight arms.

WALKOUTS

Stand with your feet hip-width apart. Bend forward from the hips and touch your hands to the floor. Walk your hands away from your body until you reach a plank position, keeping your legs as straight as possible. Slowly walk your hands back towards your feet and return to a standing position. Repeat.

TOE TOUCHES WITH TORSO TWISTS

Stand with your feet wider than hip-width apart. Keep your legs straight and bend forward from the hips. Twist to the left and take your right arm to your left foot, lifting your left arm behind you. Twist to the right and take your left arm to your right foot and your right arm behind you, rotating from the torso. Repeat.

LOWER BODY

REVERSE LUNGES WITH A TWIST

Stand with your feet hip-width apart. Take one leg behind you and lower down into a lunge with your knees both forming 90-degree angles. At the same time, lift your arms above your head and lean to the opposite side, feeling the stretch down your hip. Return to standing and repeat on the other side.

SIDE LUNGES

Stand with your feet hip-width apart. Take a step out to the side and bend the outside leg to form a 90-degree angle, with toes pointing forward. Drop down into a side lunge and feel the stretch in the inside of the lengthened leg. Return to standing and repeat on the other side.

LEG SWINGS

Stand with your feet hip-width apart. Hold on to a stable object to your side and swing the outside leg backwards and forwards, keeping your core stable and moving from the hip. Try to increase the range of motion with each swing. Repeat on the other side.

GLUTE ACTIVATION ROUTINE

You're probably reading those words and thinking 'What on earth!?' Let me explain. Glute activation is an essential part of my warm-up routine. When you sit at a desk all day, your bum cheeks (your glute muscles!) get sleepy. You aren't activating them, and you know the saying: if you don't use it, you lose it. As a result, your glutes can become weaker than the surrounding muscles, which can lead to those other muscles (such as your quadriceps, the muscles on the fronts of your thighs) being used to compensate. This can lead to injuries and imbalances in the long term. That is why it is absolutely essential to do glute activation prior to any exercise in which the glutes may come into play. Put simply, this involves a technique which 'wakes up' your glutes and opens up the connection between your brain and your muscles, preparing them to do some work. As a result, you recruit them during exercise and they strengthen and grow. This not only leads to a reduced risk of injury and improved performance in the gym but also helps to build a peachy booty!

My favourite way to activate my glutes is through the use of a small looped resistance band. The more advanced you become, the thicker the band needs to be. Here are my top three moves:

Top tip: These can also be used at the end of leg workouts for additional booty building!

WALKS

1. Pop the band around your legs, just above your knees. Take a high squat position, keeping your shoulders back and core tight.
2. Take a small step to the side, pulling from the knee and staying in the high squat (no bouncing up and down!). Take a few more steps and then go in the opposite direction. Your glutes will be on fire!

HIP THRUSTS

1. Pop the band around your legs, just above your knees, and lie down on the floor with your knees bent and feet planted.
2. Push your knees out to the sides so there is tension on the band. Keep this tension as you lift your hips towards the sky by pushing through your heels. Squeeze your glutes at the top of the movement. Return to the starting position with your knees keeping tension on the band the whole time. Repeat.

SQUATS

1. Pop the band around your legs, just above your knees. Place your feet hip-width apart and gently push your knees slightly outwards so there is tension on the band.
2. Sit back and down into a squat position, keeping your knees pushed out and your chest upright. Extend back up to a standing position by pushing through your heels. Repeat.

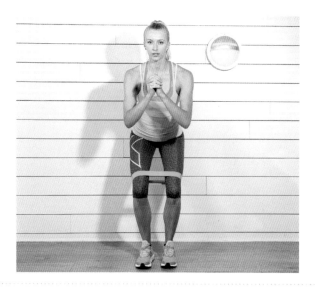
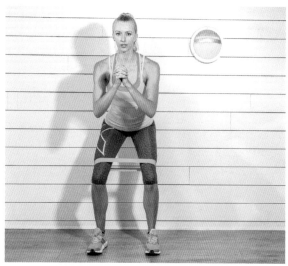
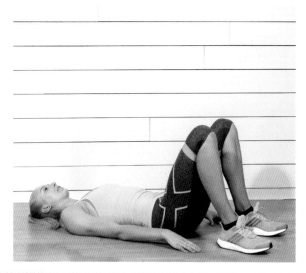
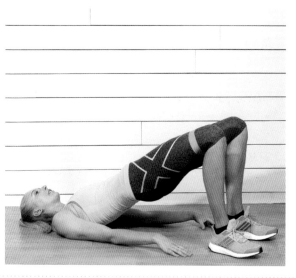
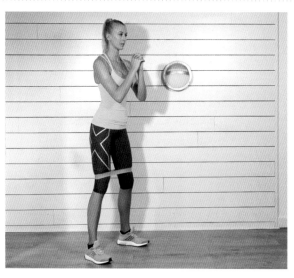
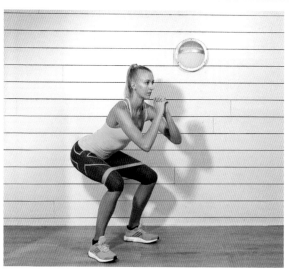

THE COOL DOWN

After every workout you need to cool down appropriately. As you perform contraction after contraction during your workout, your muscles are left in a shortened state. To cool down I recommend using a range of static stretches targeting the muscles you used (consult a personal trainer or sports expert if you are in any doubt over how to stretch safely, without risk of injury). These help to relax your muscles, restore them to their resting length and even improve flexibility. Stretching also helps to reduce the risk of injury, improve blood circulation and correct poor posture. Plus, spending 10 minutes stretching can calm your mind and provide a much-needed mental break.

When you cool down, hold each stretch for a minimum of 30 seconds to really feel the results. Don't stretch absent-mindedly either; make sure you're consciously trying to relax and breathe out as you stretch a little bit further every time. If you've been doing high-intensity cardio, be sure to reduce your heart rate before you go into stretching. The best way to do this is to engage in some lower-intensity movement, such as walking, for 5 minutes. Ensure that you do at least one stretch which targets each muscle group. You can use the following list as a starting point.

① SHOULDERS (DELTOIDS)

② CHEST (PECTORALS)

③ BICEPS

④ OBLIQUES

⑤ ABDOMINALS ('ABS')

⑥ HIP FLEXORS

⑦ HIP ADDUCTORS

⑧ QUADRICEPS ('QUADS')

⑨ TRAPEZIUS ('TRAPS')

⑩ RHOMBOIDS ('UNDER TRAPS')

⑪ LATISSIMUS DORSI ('LATS')

⑫ TRICEPS

⑬ ERECTOR SPINAE

⑭ GLUTEALS ('GLUTES')

⑮ HAMSTRINGS

⑯ CALVES

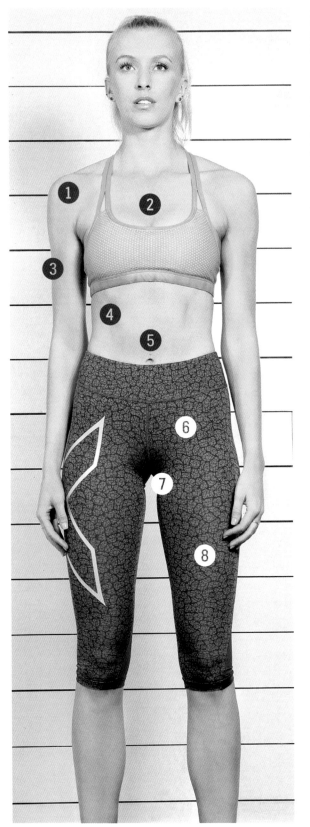
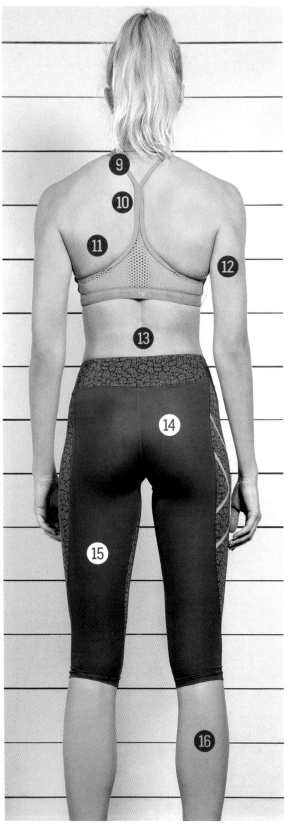

BEGINNERS

If you're totally new to resistance training and don't have a gym membership, these workouts are for you. They focus on straight sets of key exercises for each body part to ensure every muscle is worked effectively. These shouldn't take any longer than 30–40 minutes and all you need is a set of dumbbells.

BEGINNERS UPPER BODY

3 SETS OF 10—12 REPS*

Areas targeted: shoulders, triceps, biceps, back, chest and core.

*COMPLETE ALL SETS OF ONE EXERCISE BEFORE MOVING ON TO THE NEXT

FLOOR SHOULDER PRESS

1. Sit on the floor against a wall with your legs straight out in front of you, pressing your lower back into the wall the whole time.

2. Place your dumbbells at shoulder height with your palms facing forwards. Push the dumbbells upwards until they touch at the top. Lower to the starting position and repeat.

BENT-OVER ROW

1. Bend your knees slightly and bring your torso forwards, keeping your back straight. Hold the dumbbells in front of you with your palms facing inwards.

2. Bend your arms and move the dumbbells to your sides, keeping your elbows close to your body. Squeeze your back at the top of the movement. Lower to the starting position and repeat.

FLOOR CHEST PRESS

1. Lying flat on the floor with your legs bent, bring the dumbbells to either side of your chest with your arms bent.

2. Exhale and extend your arms upwards using your chest and touch the dumbbells together. Squeeze your chest at the top of the movement. Lower back to the starting position with control. Repeat.

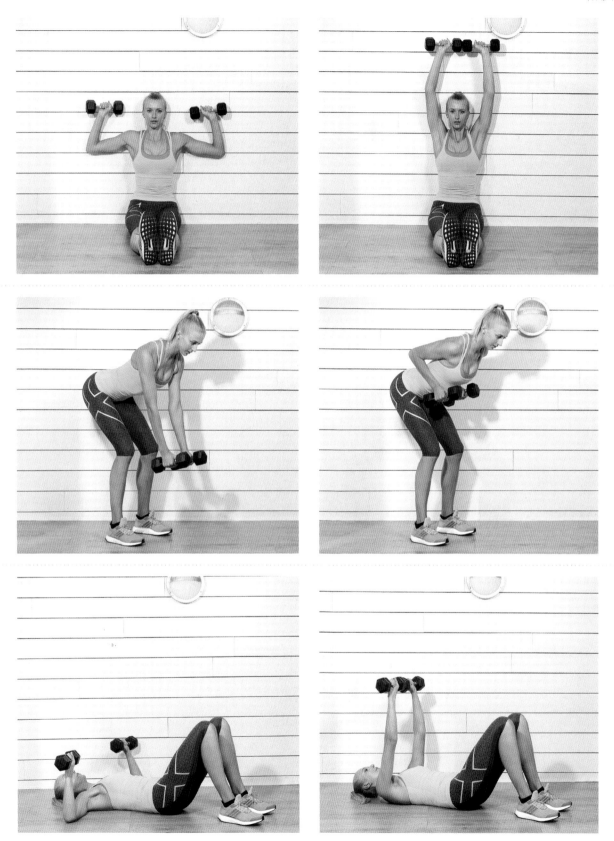

ALTERNATING BICEP CURLS

1. In a standing position with feet hip-width apart, hold the dumbbells by your sides with your shoulders pulled back and your core engaged.

2. Lift one hand, keeping your elbow tight to your side, and curl the weight up until your palm faces you. Lower back to the starting position with control. Repeat with the opposite arm.

LYING TRICEP EXTENSIONS

1. Lying on the floor with your lower back pushed into the ground, hold a weight in each hand and lift your arms above your head so that they're pointing straight up into the air with your palms facing each other.

2. Keeping your elbows stable, slowly bend your arms so as to lower the weights towards the floor over your head. Extend your arms back to the top of the movement and repeat.

MOUNTAIN CLIMBERS

1. Start in a high plank position with your hands beneath your shoulders.

2. Bend one leg and pull it forwards towards your elbow and then lower it back to the starting position. Repeat with the opposite leg, keeping your core engaged and back straight. Do this movement **very** slowly and with control. Your whole core will be shaking in no time!

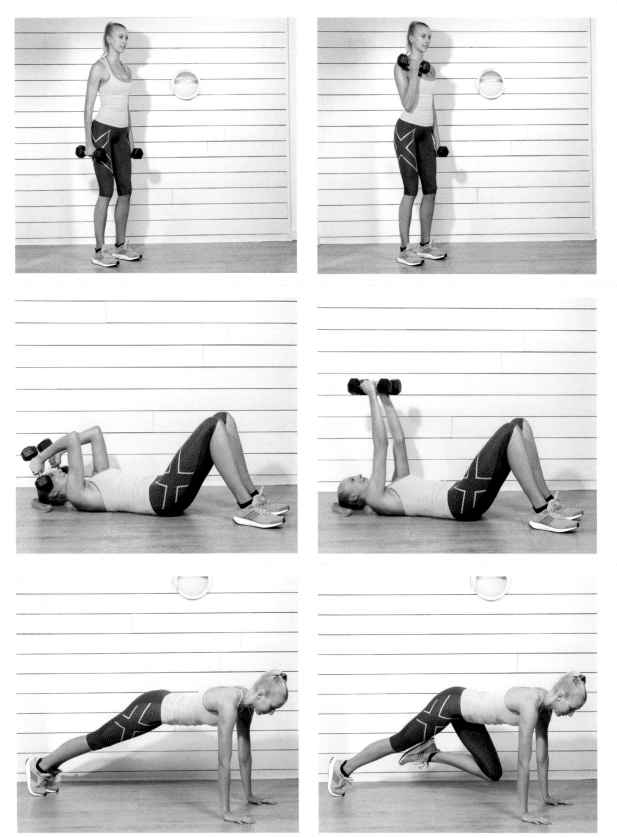

BEGINNERS LOWER BODY

3 SETS OF 10—12 REPS*

Areas targeted:
glutes, quads, hamstrings,
calves and core.

*COMPLETE ALL SETS OF
ONE EXERCISE BEFORE
MOVING ON TO THE NEXT

GOBLET SQUATS

1. Stand with your feet a little wider than hip-width apart and toes ever so slightly pointing outwards. Hold the weights to your chest.

2. Squat down until your knees are at a right-angle, sitting back into the movement and ensuring your knees don't travel over your toes. Keep your chest up and back straight. Return to a standing position and repeat.

BULGARIAN SPLIT SQUATS

1. Stand with one foot on the floor and another on an elevated surface behind you, holding the dumbbells by your sides.

2. Keeping your chest upright, bend your front leg and lower yourself back and down until your front knee is at a right-angle, ensuring your knees don't travel over your toes. Push up through your front heel and return to the starting position. Do all 10-12 reps on one leg before switching sides.

WALKING LUNGES

1. Stand with your feet shoulder-width apart and with a dumbbell in each hand.

2. Step forwards with one leg into a long stride and lower into a lunge, bending both knees and keeping your posture upright while ensuring your knees don't travel over your toes. Drive through your front heel to return to standing, then repeat by stepping forwards with the opposite leg into another stride. Repeat.

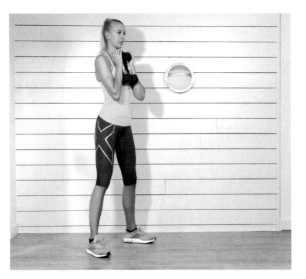

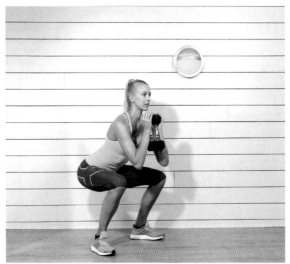

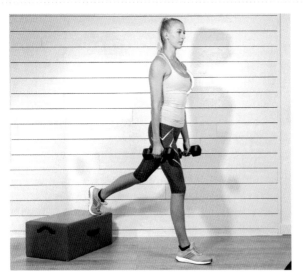

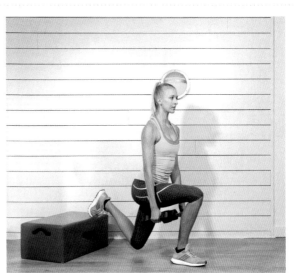

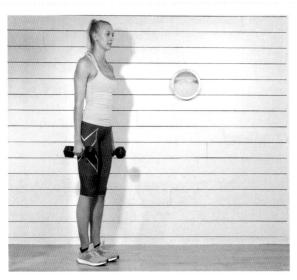

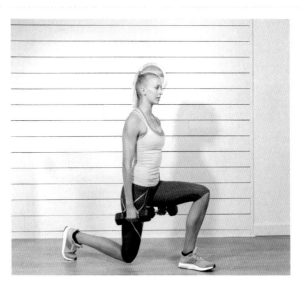

ROMANIAN DEADLIFTS

1. Stand with your feet shoulder-width apart and hold the dumbbells in front of you, palms facing you. Bend your knees ever so slightly and hinge forwards from the hips, keeping your back straight.

2. Lower the weights towards the floor, keeping them close to your legs, and feel the pull down your hamstrings. Return to the starting position, squeezing your glutes at the top. Repeat.

STEP-UPS

1. Stand with a raised platform in front of you and dumbbells held by your sides. Place one foot on the platform.

2. Push up through the heel of the foot on the platform to lift yourself off the floor and come completely onto the step. Lower the same leg back to the floor with control and repeat. Keep the working leg on the platform until all reps are completed before switching sides.

DUMBBELL GLUTE BRIDGE

1. Lying flat on the floor with your legs bent, hold the dumbbells on your hips.

2. Pushing through your heels, extend your hips towards the sky and squeeze your glutes together at the top of the movement. Return to the starting position with control. Repeat.

Top tip: After you have completed all the reps, hold yourself at the top of the movement and squeeze your bum cheeks hard for 15–20 seconds to get a **serious** booty burn! Ouch!

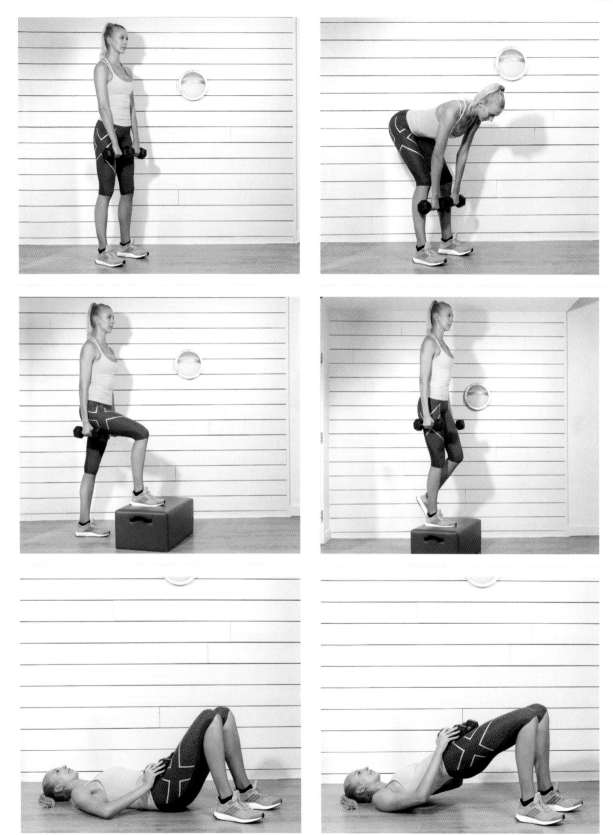

BEGINNERS FULL BODY

3 SETS OF 10—12 REPS*

Areas targeted:
everythaaaang!

*COMPLETE ALL SETS OF
ONE EXERCISE BEFORE
MOVING ON TO THE NEXT

SQUAT AND PRESS

1. Stand with your feet a little wider than hip-width apart and your toes ever so slightly pointing outwards. Hold the weights at shoulder height with your palms facing inwards.

2. Lower down into a squat position, keeping your chest upright. As you return to a standing position, in a smooth movement push the weights up above you into a shoulder press with your arms extended overhead. As you lower your arms, return to a squat position. Repeat.

CURTSEY LUNGE WITH CURL

1. Stand with your feet hip-width apart and dumbbells by your sides.

2. Step back and to the side in a diagonal movement, crossing the moving leg behind the static leg, and lower into a lunge until your front knee is at a right-angle. As you step into the lunge, curl both arms upwards and bring your palms to your chest with your elbows tight to your sides. As you step out of the lunge (returning to the starting point), lower your arms back to your sides. Repeat on the opposite leg.

PUSH-UPS

1. On the floor, come into a high plank position with your hands directly below your shoulders and feet together.

2. Bend your arms until your elbows are at a right-angle, lowering your chest towards the floor and keeping your core engaged and back straight. Straighten your arms to return to the starting position and repeat.

Top tip: If this is too challenging then this movement can be done on your knees. Just ensure there is a straight line from your head to your knees.

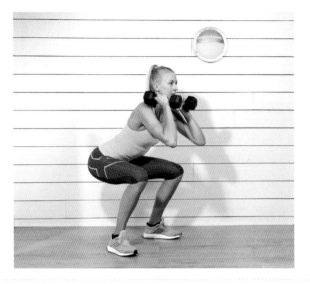

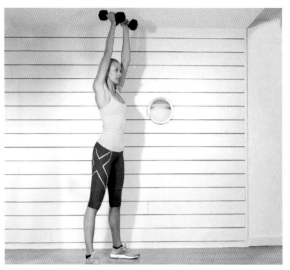

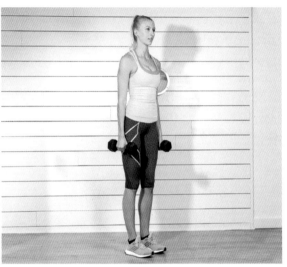

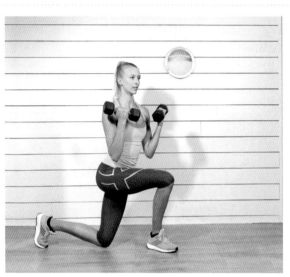

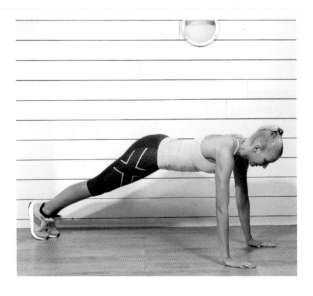

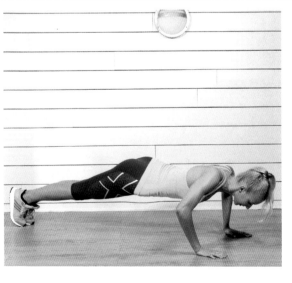

SINGLE-ARM ROWS

1. Hold a dumbbell in one hand and place your other hand on a stable raised platform at around knee height, softening your knees, leaning your body forwards and keeping your back straight.

2. Allow the weight to naturally hang below you, then bend your arm to pull the weight to your torso, keeping your elbow tight to your body and squeezing your back at the top of the movement. Lower to the starting position and do all reps on one arm before switching sides.

BENT-OVER TRICEP EXTENSIONS

1. In a standing position, bend your knees slightly and lean your torso forwards, keeping your back straight. Keep your arms close to your body with your palms facing inwards.

2. Squeezing your triceps, extend your arms backwards until they are straight and squeeze your triceps at the top of the movement. Lower back to the starting position with control. Repeat.

RUSSIAN TWISTS

1. Sit on the floor with your knees bent and feet flat on the ground. Hold a dumbbell out in front of you. Keep your back straight and lean back.

2. From here, twist your upper body and core to one side until your arms are parallel to the floor. Return to the starting position and repeat on the other side. That is one rep.

Top tip: Your heels can be lifted off the floor for a more challenging exercise, as pictured.

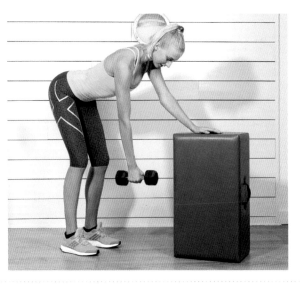

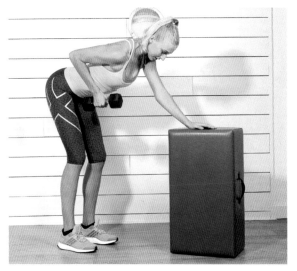

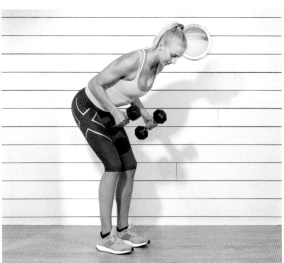

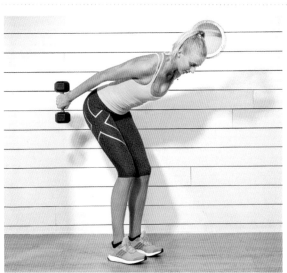

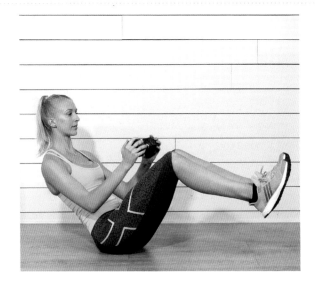

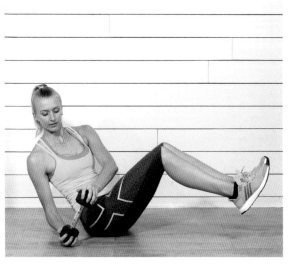

ADVANCED

These workouts use more complex and challenging movements which require gym-based equipment. Techniques such as drop sets are used to push your body in new ways! These workouts are for those of you who have been lifting for a while and feel comfortable with this form of training. Use these exercises if you have built up a base level of strength and mobility and are up for a challenge. Bring on the burn!

ADVANCED UPPER BODY

3 SETS OF 8—12 REPS*

Areas targeted:
shoulders, triceps, biceps,
back, chest and core.

*COMPLETE ALL SETS OF
ONE EXERCISE BEFORE
MOVING ON TO THE NEXT

DUMBBELL SHOULDER PRESS DROP SETS

1. Sitting on a bench, place the dumbbells at shoulder height with your palms facing forwards.

2. Push the dumbbells upwards until they touch at the top. Lower to the starting position and repeat. After you have completed one set, immediately reduce the weight by about 50 percent and do another set. Feel the burn!

BARBELL ROW WITH HOLD

1. Stand with your feet hip-width apart, bend your knees and lower your torso towards the floor, keeping your back straight.

2. Holding a barbell in front of you with an overhand grip, bend your arms and lift the barbell towards you. Keep your elbows close to your sides and squeeze your shoulder blades together at the top of the movement. Hold it here for a moment, then lower the barbell to the starting position and repeat.

ECCENTRIC PUSH-UPS

1. On the floor, come into a high plank position with your hands directly below your shoulders and feet together.

2. **Very slowly**, bend your arms until your elbows are at a right-angle, lowering your chest towards the floor and keeping your core engaged and back straight. This eccentric phase of the movement should take a minimum of 3-5 seconds. Straighten your arms to return to the starting position. Repeat.

Top tip: If this is too challenging then this movement can be done on your knees. Just ensure there is a straight line from your head to your knees.

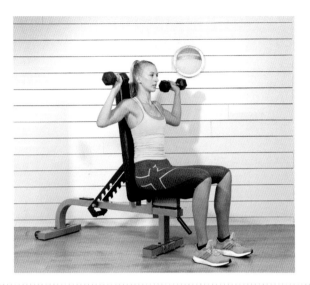
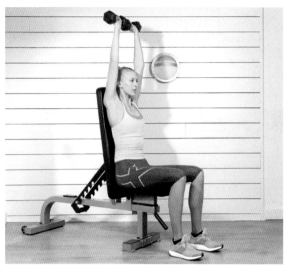
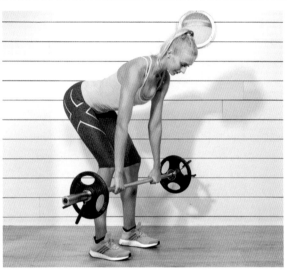
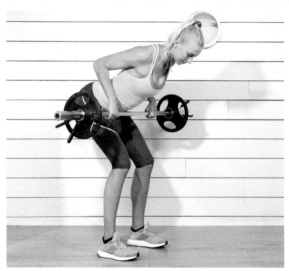
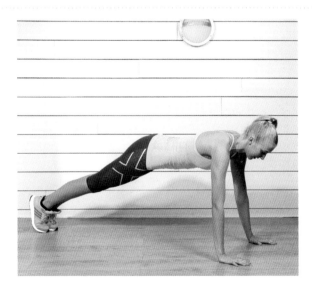
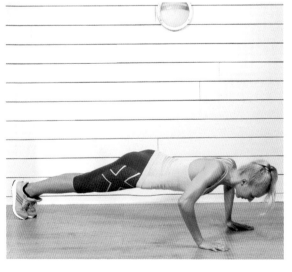

DUMBBELL CLOSE-GRIP BENCH PRESS

1. Lying flat on your back on a bench, bring the dumbbells together in front of you with your palms facing inwards.

2. Exhale and extend your arms upwards using your chest and triceps and squeezing at the top of the movement. Lower back to the starting position with control. Repeat.

DUMBBELL HAMMER CURLS

1. In a standing position with your feet hip-width apart, hold the dumbbells by your sides with your palms facing inwards. Keep your shoulders pulled back and core engaged.

2. Lift one hand, keeping your elbow tight to your side, and curl the weight up, keeping your palm facing inwards. Lower back to the starting position with control. Repeat with the opposite arm.

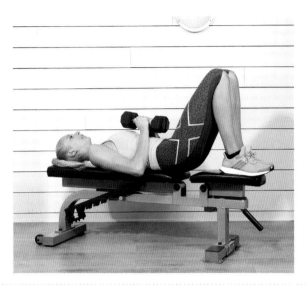
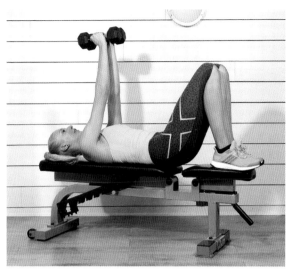
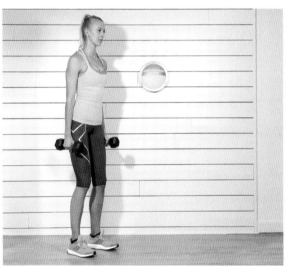
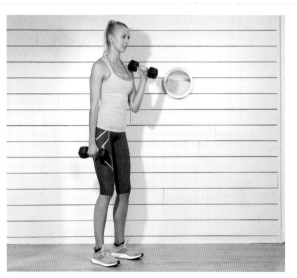

ADVANCED LOWER BODY

3 SETS OF 8—12 REPS*

Areas targeted:
glutes, quads, hamstrings,
calves and core.

*COMPLETE ALL SETS OF
ONE EXERCISE BEFORE
MOVING ON TO THE NEXT

BARBELL SQUATS

1. Start in a standing position with a barbell across your back, feet hip-width apart and toes slightly pointed out.

2. Sit back and down into a squat position, keeping your torso upright and back straight and avoiding letting your knees travel over your toes. From the bottom of the movement, reverse the motion by pushing up through your heels and straightening your legs. Squeeze your glutes and push your hips slightly forwards at the top of the movement.

BARBELL SUMO DEADLIFTS

1. Standing behind a barbell with your feet wide and toes pointing outwards, bend at the knees and hips to grab it with both hands with your arms directly below your shoulders. Engage your core, lengthen your arms, relax your neck and lower your hips to sit back, ensuring your back isn't rounded.

2. Drive up through your heels and extend through your hips and knees, keeping the bar close to your body and squeezing your glutes at the top of the movement. Reverse the movement to return the weight to the ground.

BARBELL HIP THRUSTS

1. Sit on the ground with your back against a bench and your feet hip-width apart, with a barbell on your hips. You can pop a cushion or pad underneath it for comfort.

2. Lean back against the bench, resting on your shoulder blades. Drive through your feet and extend your hips vertically, lifting the bar. At the top of the movement be sure to squeeze your glutes and not overextend your lower back. Return to the starting position with control. Repeat.

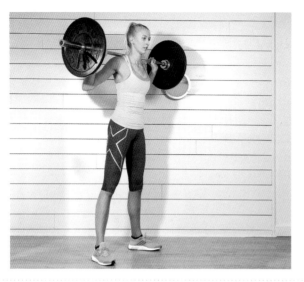

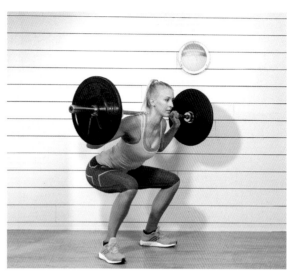

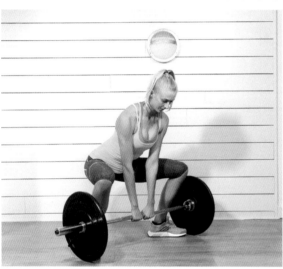

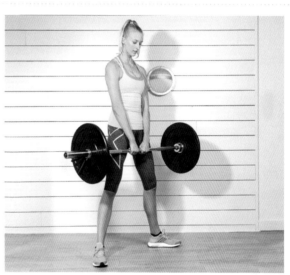

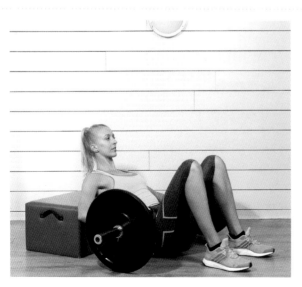

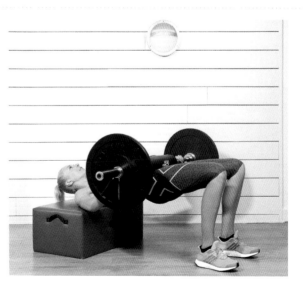

LEG PRESS

1. Add your desired weight to the leg press. Sit down in the machine and place your legs on the platform in front of you shoulder-width apart. Push your legs away from you until they are fully extended, avoiding locking your knees.

2. Slowly bend your legs and lower the platform towards yourself until your legs form a right-angle. Repeat.

Top tip: You can change your foot position to target different elements of the leg. For example, a narrow stance targets the quadriceps and a wide stance targets the hamstrings and glutes.

STATIC LUNGE

1. Start in a long stride position with one foot in front of the other and the weights held by your sides.

2. Bend both legs to form two right-angles and lower yourself towards the floor. Keeping your torso upright, extend your legs to bring yourself back to the starting position. Repeat.

BALL HAMSTRING CURLS

1. Lying on the floor, place your heels on top of a Swiss ball and place your hands by your sides. Lift your hips off the floor so there is a straight line from your toes to your shoulders.

2. From here, bend your knees and lift your hips towards the sky, at the same time rolling the ball in towards yourself. Then slowly roll your legs back out to the starting position, lowering your hips back so they form a straight line with the rest of your body. Repeat.

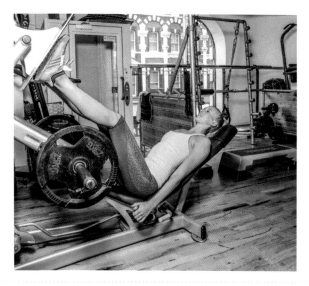
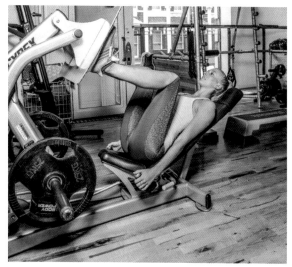

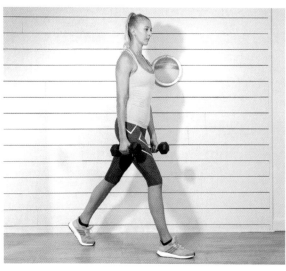
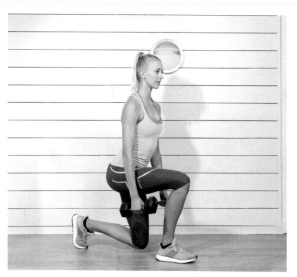

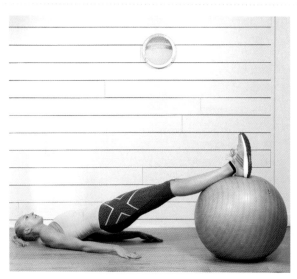
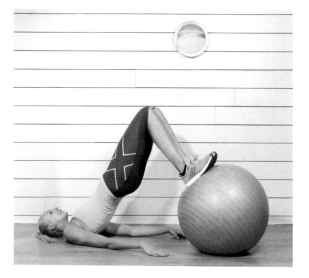

ADVANCED FULL BODY

3 SETS OF 8—12 REPS*

Areas targeted: everythaaaang!

*COMPLETE ALL SETS OF ONE EXERCISE BEFORE MOVING ON TO THE NEXT

DEADLIFTS

1. Stand behind a bar with your feet hip-width apart. Bend at the hips and grip the bar at shoulder width. Lower your hips and flex your knees so that your shins are touching the bar. Keep your chest and torso upright, back straight and neck relaxed.

2. Drive through your heels to move the weight upwards. After the bar passes your knees, pull your shoulders back, push your hips forwards into the bar and squeeze your glutes. Return to the starting position by bending your knees and hips, keeping your core engaged the whole time. Repeat.

CURTSEY LUNGES AND SIDE LUNGES

1. Stand with your feet hip-width apart and dumbbells by your sides. Step back and to the side in a diagonal movement, crossing the moving leg behind the static leg, and lower into a lunge until your front knee is at a right-angle.

2. Step up out of the lunge (returning to the starting point) and then take a big stride with the same leg out to the side and lower into a side lunge, keeping your chest upright. Return to the starting position and repeat. Do all the reps on one leg before changing to the other.

DUMBELL SUMO SQUAT INTO CURL AND PRESS

1. Standing with your feet wider than hip-width apart and toes pointing outwards, hold the dumbbells in your hands directly in front of you. Lower down into a sumo squat, pushing your knees wide and letting the weights hang down, keeping your torso upright.

2. As you extend out of the sumo squat, curl the weights up to your chest and then press them overhead by extending them into a shoulder press. Then return your arms to the starting position, by reversing the movement. Repeat.

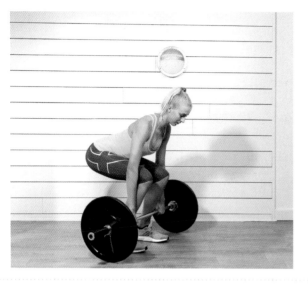

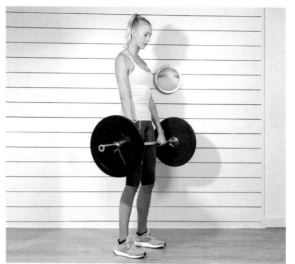

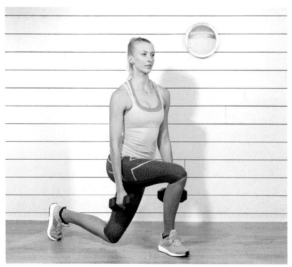

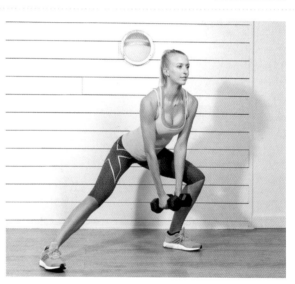

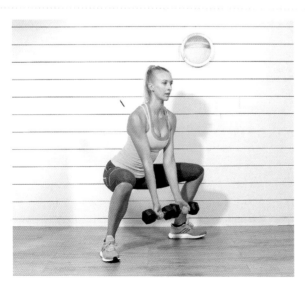

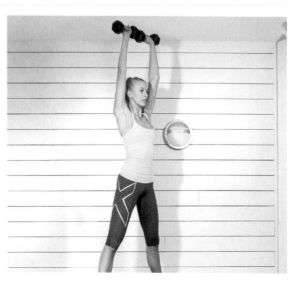

PUSH-UP INTO RENEGADE ROW

1. Start in a plank position with your hands on two dumbbells. Lower yourself towards the floor into a press-up, keeping your back straight. Extend back into a plank position.

2. From here, keeping your core engaged and stable, lift one dumbbell up to your side, keeping your elbow tight to your side, and then lower it back to the floor. Repeat with the opposite arm. That is one complete rep.

RESISTANCE BAND TRICEP DIPS

1. Place a resistance band over a set of dip bars. Place your knees onto it and hold your body at arm's length above the bars.

2. Lower yourself downwards by bending your arms until a right-angle is formed. Keep your torso upright and elbows close to your body. Push yourself back up to the starting position.

SWISS BALL ROLL-OUTS

1. Kneel in front of a Swiss ball and place your forearms on it.

2. Lean forwards and roll the ball out in front of you, keeping your core engaged and back straight. Go as far as you can before pushing back up to the starting position.

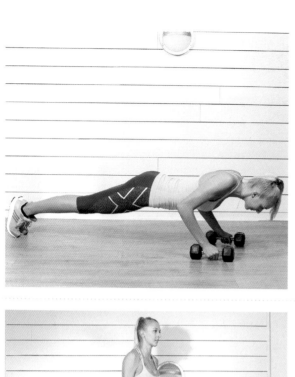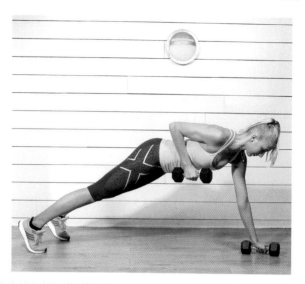

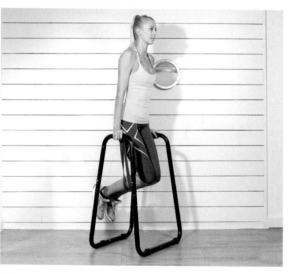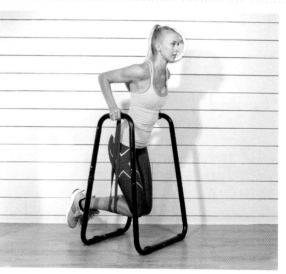

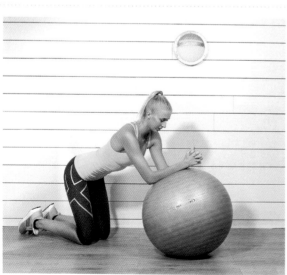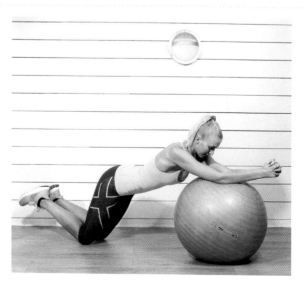

PUTTING IT ALL TOGETHER

GETTING STARTED

Now that you have these workouts, you're probably wondering how to get started with them! Here is my four-step guide:

1. Decide whether you're a beginner or an advanced weight lifter. This will depend on your previous experience, your confidence and your access to equipment. If you work out at home, I highly recommend investing in a selection of dumbbells and kettle bells which are a variety of weights. This will mean that you can continuously progress your workouts.

2. Decide how many times you would like to do weighted workouts per week and use this to guide how you split up your training. For beginners I recommend doing weights one to three times a week and focusing on upper, lower and full-body workouts as opposed to more detailed splits. This will ease you into it and give you time to explore other forms of exercise too. Then as you advance (and fall in love with weights!) you can take on more resistance workouts per week and a more advanced split if you would like to (more on that later).

3. Get started! Pick up those dumbbells and challenge yourself. I promise you will be hooked sooner than you think. If you're wondering what weight to use, there is no single right answer. It totally depends on your body's strength, and you will have to go

through a bit of trial and error on your first workout to find out how much you can lift. My recommendation is to find a weight which you really struggle to lift for the last couple of reps.

4. Keep progressing and switch it up. Every single week you should be trying to increase your reps or weight on each exercise, to ensure your body consistently gets stronger. I also recommend changing up your workouts every 6-8 weeks by incorporating new moves and trying different routines and combinations. This should help you to avoid hitting plateaus in your progress.

HOW DO YOU SWITCH IT UP?

You didn't think I was just going to give you a few workouts and leave it there, did you? Of course not. These exercises are a great starting point, but they are just that - a starting point. Quite frankly, if you just did these routines every day for the rest of your life, your body would get used to them pretty quickly and your results would slow to a halt. I don't want that to happen. I am going to equip you with all the tools you need to create endless custom workouts based on exactly what **you** want to achieve, so that you can continue to get lasting results long into the future.

First things first: let's discuss the various ways that you can progress within a given workout, including the ones I have designed for you.

Ultimately, our goal is to lift heavier weights and as a result get stronger, but how exactly do we do that? There are two key approaches:

1. Increase the number of reps you're doing with a particular weight. For example, if you're doing a shoulder press with 6 kg dumbbells one week for 8 reps, the next week try to do it for 9-10 reps and the week after go for 11-12 reps. If your goal is hypertrophy (which will be defined later), when once you hit 12 reps I recommend increasing the weight and reducing the reps back down to 8, and working up again from there.

2. Increase the weight you're lifting. This is when you keep the rep range the same but you attempt to add a small amount of weight to the exercise. For example, one week you could shoulder press 6 kg for 8 reps and the next week you could try to shoulder press 7 kg for 8 reps.

There are a whole host of other more complex ways to develop strength, but ultimately it all comes down to the basic principle of progressively overloading the muscle in one way or another. How often should you do this? As often as you can, but don't worry if you can't increase the weight or reps every week. Sometimes we just need to spend a few weeks at a certain weight or rep range before our body lets us get stronger!

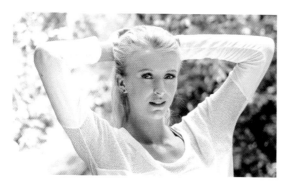

CREATING A PROGRAMME

Now you know how to progress within a workout, let's talk about creating yourself a whole new training session. I recommend that every 6-8 weeks you reassess your training, reflect on where you are with your goals, think about what you have enjoyed and decide what you would like to focus on next. You can design new workouts for yourself or change the structure or design of your current workouts, to ensure you keep on progressing. Here are the key things you need to consider when you're designing a workout.

HOW OFTEN ARE YOU GOING TO TRAIN PER WEEK?

Do you want to lift one, two, three, four or more times each week? This will determine how you split up your workouts. If you're a beginner, I recommend sticking to upper, lower and/or full-body workouts to start with. For example, if you do two weighed workouts per week, you could do one for your upper body and one for your lower body, or you could do two full-body workouts. Once you start doing four or more weighted workouts per week, you can start using more complex workout splits. Here are two examples of how you might split up your weekly workouts:

Workout 1:	legs
Workout 2:	back & biceps
Workout 3:	chest & triceps
Workout 4:	shoulders & arms

Workout 1:	legs (hamstrings & glutes dominant)
Workout 2:	legs (quads dominant)
Workout 3:	chest, shoulders & arms
Workout 4:	back & biceps

How you decide to split up your workouts is totally up to you and depends on your strengths, weaknesses, preferences and goals. If you're new to weight training, I don't recommend trying to train four or five days per week as your body will need more time to recover and repair than the body of somebody who is more used to training. Go easy on yourself. Even if you're experienced with weight training, if you have a hectic life and struggle to get to the gym, don't put pressure on yourself to train every day. It could do more harm than good. If you lift weights consistently and ensure you push yourself, train hard and keep progressing, the results will come!

WHAT ARE YOUR GOALS?

Do you want to get stronger, build up muscle tone, develop muscular endurance or a combination of all three? Your answer will determine the rep range and rest periods you should use. Here are some basic guidelines:

• For strength, do 1-6 reps and then rest for 2-4 minutes before your next set.

• For strength and hypertrophy (muscle growth and resulting improved muscle tone), do 6-8 reps and then rest for 1-2 minutes before your next set.

• For hypertrophy with some strength gains, do 8-12 reps and then rest for 1 minute before your next set.

• For endurance, do 12-15 reps (or more) and then rest for 30 seconds before your next set.

It is totally up to you which rep range you use but here are a few recommendations:

• Don't do 1-rep maxes (1 rep as heavy as possible) on a regular basis, as they are very taxing on the body and have a higher risk of injury.

• Avoid just doing endurance training as this leads to minimal strength gains.

• Pure hypertrophy training is great if you want to build muscle tone while developing some strength, and it is a great place for beginners to start.

• Once you're comfortable lifting weights, a combination of strength training and hypertrophy training is a great way to build muscle **and** get stronger! For example, I personally like to start off my workouts with a couple of key exercises for 6-8 reps to build up strength in these areas before moving on to a rep range more suited to hypertrophy, which helps to build muscle tone by increasing muscle volume.

Disclaimer: When weight training, good form is **essential.** As much as I can try to explain how to perform exercises in this book, I can't watch you in person and make sure you're doing them right. In order to avoid injury and ensure you're training correctly, I highly recommend working with a personal trainer for a few hours. Ask them to run you through all of the exercises with a focus on the squats and deadlifts, which are particularly complex.

HOW ARE YOU GOING TO STRUCTURE YOUR WORKOUT?

This totally depends on your time constraints, as well as your preferences. I personally love to do one heavy compound strength-focused movement at the beginning and then move on to three or more hypertrophy-focused exercises or supersets (pairs of exercises done back to back). Find what works for you.

• How many exercises do you want to do? Pick the key exercises you want to work on. Remember, more isn't always better. It can be just as effective to focus on four exercises for more sets as it is to do eight exercises for fewer sets.

• How many sets do you want to do per exercise? A great place to start is 3 sets of 10 reps, but don't limit yourself to that as you advance. A general rule of thumb is that the more reps you do, the fewer sets you do. For example, you might do 5 sets of 5 reps, 4 sets of 8 reps or 3 sets of 10–12 reps.

• How do you want to order the exercises? I recommend doing the most challenging compound movements (e.g., deadlifts, squats, overhead presses or pull-ups) at the beginning of a workout so that you can put enough energy into them. Then, as you tire, move into lighter isolation or accessory movements, which have a lower risk of injury.

HOW ARE YOU GOING TO CHALLENGE YOURSELF?

As a beginner, changing the exercises you do as well as the sets, reps and weights will be more than enough to change your body. However, as you advance, you can add in more complex techniques:

• Use drop sets, supersets, trisets and giant sets. These not only challenge your muscles but also are very time efficient and mean you can squeeze more out of your workout.

• Change the speed at which you execute an exercise. For example, you can elongate the eccentric phase of a movement to make a muscle spend more time under tension.

• Add in more complex exercises. For example, you can use single-leg Romanian deadlifts to challenge your stability and balance.

Don't forget that less is more. Don't try to add all of these techniques to your next workout programme as you will exhaust your resources, leaving you with fewer tools to play with and manipulate in the future. Your body only needs small incremental changes to progress. Try adding in one technique or change at a time and seeing how your body reacts.

It is important to note that these are just a handful of ways in which you can challenge your body through weighted workouts. There are so many different approaches that I wish I could cover, from periodisation to German volume training, but I simply can't fit them all into this book. Don't be afraid to read around, and never stop learning!

WHAT EXERCISES ARE YOU GOING TO DO?

Now comes the fun part: deciding on the exercises you want to include in your workouts! Here are my top picks for each body part, excluding the moves included in the structured workouts found earlier in the book.

SHOULDERS

Top tip: There are three heads to the shoulder — the anterior (front), medial (middle) and posterior (back) — all of which need to be trained to avoid imbalances. This combination of exercises hits all three.

BARBELL PRESS

1. In a seated position with a rack in front of you, grip the barbell with both hands and hold it below your chin with your arms bent.

2. Pushing your lower back into the seat, extend your arms overhead and push the barbell above you. Return to the starting position and repeat.

ARNOLD PRESS

1. In a seated position, hold a pair of dumbbells in front of your chest with your palms facing you.

2. Pushing your lower back into the seat, extend your arms overhead and twist the dumbbells so your palms face away from you in one smooth movement. Return to the starting position and repeat.

FACE PULLS

1. Facing a cable machine with a rope or dual handles attached, start with straight arms and pull the weight towards your face, simultaneously moving your hands apart.

2. Keep your arms parallel to the ground and squeeze your upper back at the top of the movement. Slowly return to the starting position and repeat.

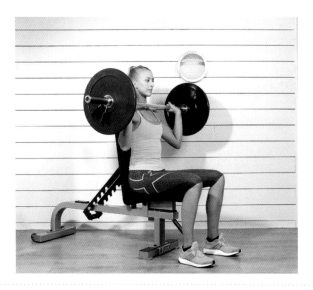

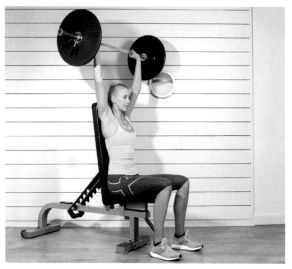

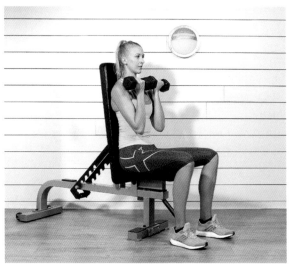

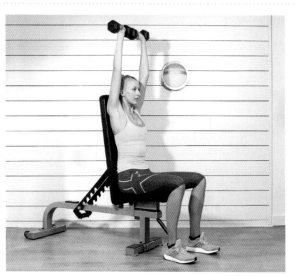

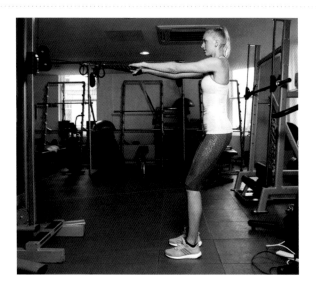

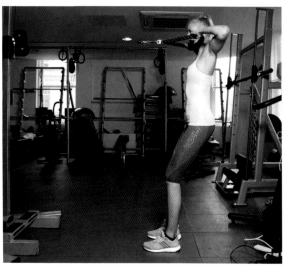

TRICEPS

BARBELL SKULL-CRUSHERS

1. In a lying position with your lower back pushed into the bench, hold a barbell in your hands and lift your arms above your head so they are at a right-angle to your body.

2. Keeping your elbows stable, slowly bend your arms and lower the barbell towards the floor over your head. Extend your arms back to the top of the movement and repeat.

Top tip: You can have your feet on the ground or on the bench, depending on how you feel most comfortable and stable.

CABLE PUSH-DOWNS

1. Standing in front of a cable machine with a flat bar attached, hold the bar with your hands shoulder-width apart with an overhand grip. Lock your elbows to your sides and start with your arms at right-angles.

2. Extend your arms into a straight position while pulling the cable downwards. Squeeze your triceps at the bottom of the movement and then slowly release back to a right-angle position. Repeat.

SEATED OVERHEAD EXTENSIONS

1. In a seated position, push your lower back into the bench. Raise a dumbbell overhead and hold it with both hands.

2. Slowly bend at the elbows and lower the weight behind you, keeping your arms stable. Then extend your arms using your triceps and push the weight back above you to returning to the starting position. Repeat.

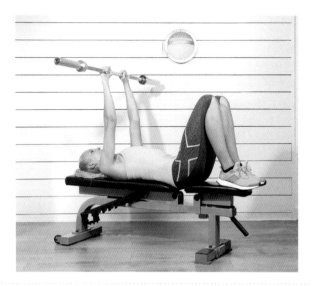 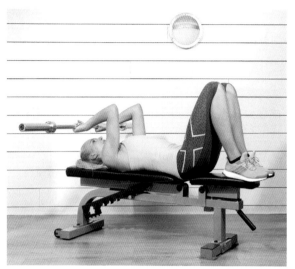

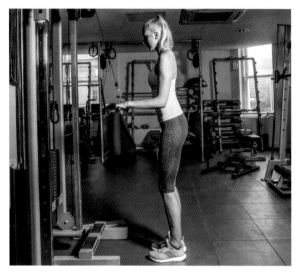 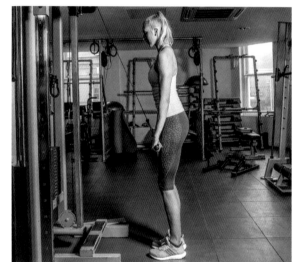

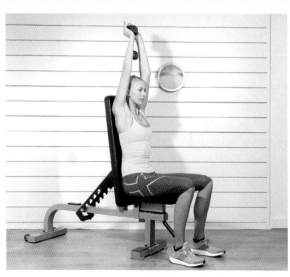 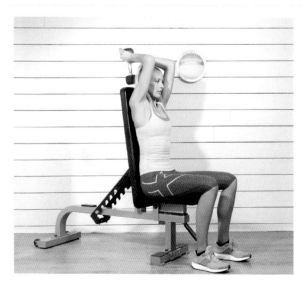

BICEPS

BARBELL CURLS

1. In a standing position, hold a barbell in front of you with an underhand grip. Keep your elbows locked to your sides, roll your shoulders back and engage your core.

2. Bend at the elbows and bring the barbell up towards your chest, pulling from the biceps. Slowly release back to the starting position, avoiding completely locking out your arms at the bottom. Repeat.

INCLINE CURLS

1. In a seated position on an incline bench, hold a dumbbell in each hand and allow your arms to hang beside you with palms facing inwards.

2. From here, curl your arms upwards, keeping your elbows tight to your sides and twisting so your palms face your chest. Slowly release back to the starting position with control. Repeat.

CABLE CURLS

1. Standing in front of a cable machine with a flat bar attached, place your hands shoulder-width apart with an underhand grip. Lock your elbows to your sides and start with your arms extended.

2. Bend your arms and pull the bar up towards your chest, squeezing your biceps at the top of the movement. Slowly release back to the starting position. Repeat.

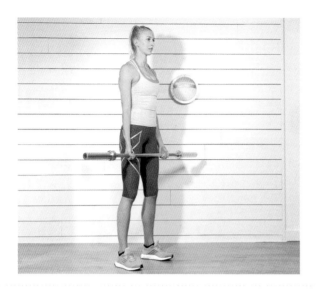
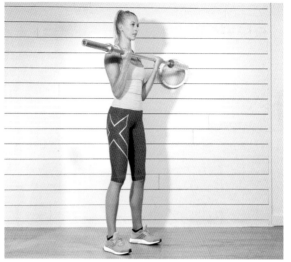

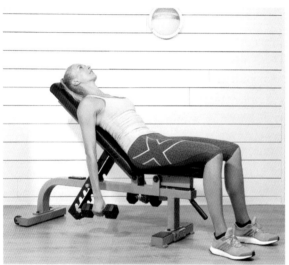
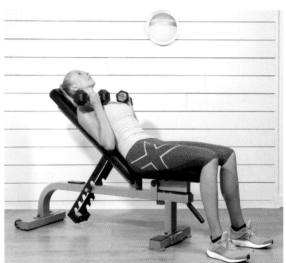

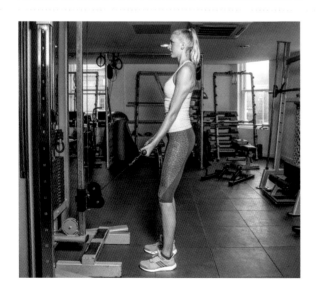
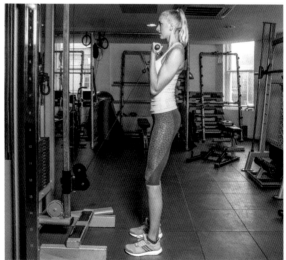

CHEST

DUMBBELL CHEST FLYES

1. Lying on a bench, extend your arms above you so the dumbbells are directly over your chest with your palms facing each other.

2. With a slight bend in your arms, move them outwards towards the floor, opening up the chest and feeling a stretch across it. Then raise your arms and bring them back together above you. Repeat.

DUMBBELL INCLINE PRESS

1. In a seated position on an incline bench, hold the dumbbells next to your chest with your arms bent.

2. Extend your arms, push the dumbbells above you and bring them together so that they touch, squeezing your chest at the top of the movement. Lower back to the starting position and repeat.

STAGGERED PUSH-UPS

1. Start in a high plank position. Place one hand slightly in front of you and one hand slightly further back.

2. Bend your arms and lower yourself into a push-up position, moving your chest towards the floor. Extend back to the top of the movement and switch the position of your arms. Repeat.

Top tip: This can be done on the knees if required.

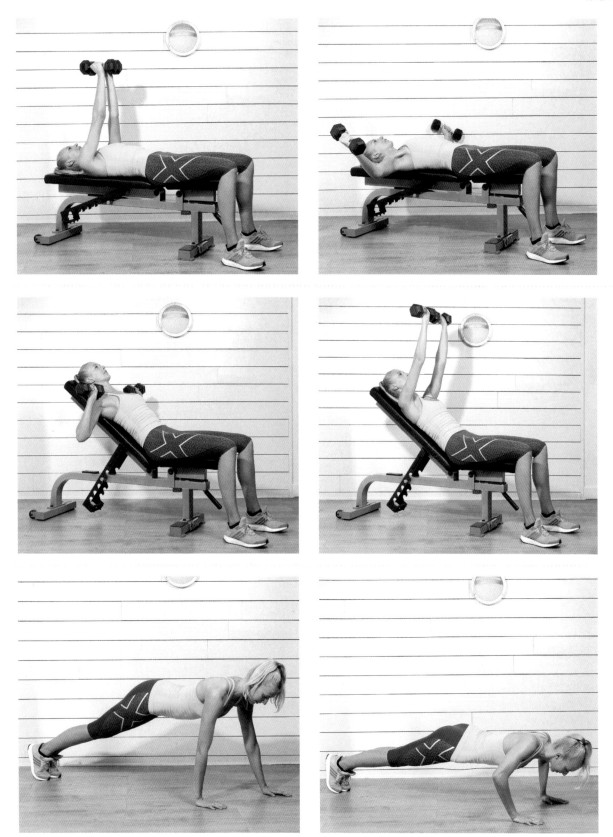

BACK

T-BAR ROWS

1. This is my favourite back exercise! Start by setting up a T-bar with a narrow handle (a trainer can help you do this). Then stand over it and bend down, keeping your back straight, and pick up the weight.

2. Set yourself into a bent-over position with your core engaged, your back straight and your arms extended in front of you. Pull the bar towards you, bending your arms and keeping your elbows tight to your sides. Squeeze your back at the top of the movement and lower back to the starting position. Repeat.

LAT PULL-DOWNS

1. This is a classic. Sit down in the lat pull-down machine and grip the long bar attachment at the widest point with an overhand grip.

2. Keeping your body stable, pull the bar down to just below your chin, squeezing your lats at the bottom of the movement. Extend your arms and return to the starting position. Repeat.

Top tip: This exercise can be performed with your hands at wide, middle or narrow grip points and with overhand or underhand grips to challenge your back in new ways!

STRAIGHT-ARM PULL-DOWNS

1. Standing in front of a cable machine with a flat bar attached, place your hands on the bar shoulder-width apart with an overhand grip. Step back and bend from the hips, keeping your back straight and arms extended overhead, gripping the bar.

2. From here, engage your core and keep your arms completely straight as you pull the bar down towards your legs. Squeeze your lats at the bottom of the movement and then slowly return to the starting position. Repeat.

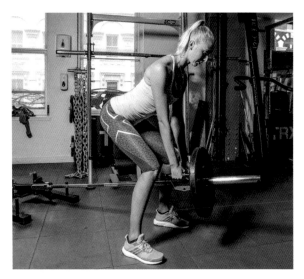
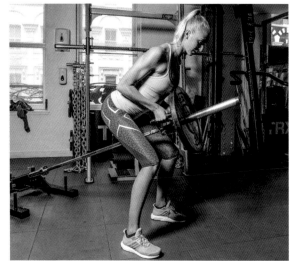
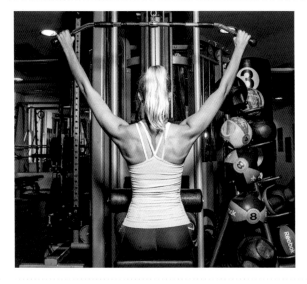
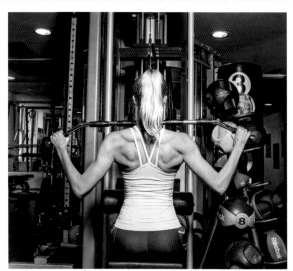
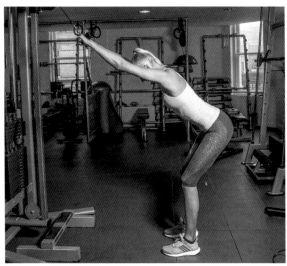
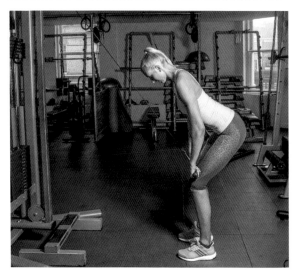

LEGS

GOOD MORNINGS

1. With a barbell on your back, stand with your feet hip-width apart and toes pointing forwards.

2. Soften your knees and hinge forwards from your hips, relaxing your neck, keeping your back straight and lowering your upper body towards the floor. Once your torso is parallel to the floor, pull up through your hamstrings to return to the starting position and squeeze your glutes at the top. Repeat.

Top tip: Good mornings are a great exercise to support good posture.

SINGLE-LEG ROMANIAN DEADLIFTS

1. Holding a dumbbell in one hand, stand on the opposite leg and lift the other leg off the floor.

2. Softening the knee of your straight leg and hinging from the hips, lean forwards, keeping the weight close to your body and back straight. Feel the stretch down the back of your legs and then pull up using your glutes and hamstrings. Squeeze your booty at the top. Do all the reps on one leg before you switch sides.

FRONT SQUAT WITH KETTLE BELLS

1. Standing with feet hip-width apart and toes pointed ever so slightly outwards, pick up the kettle bells and rest them on your upper arms, keeping your arms parallel to the floor.

2. Keeping your chest high, sit back and down into a squat position with your knees at right-angles. Then push up through your heels to return to the starting position. Repeat.

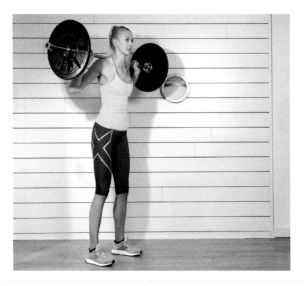

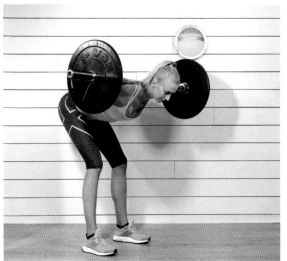

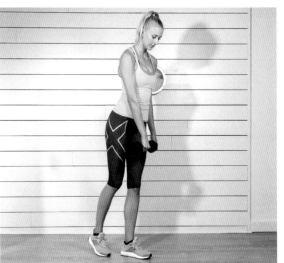

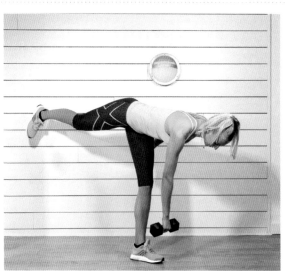

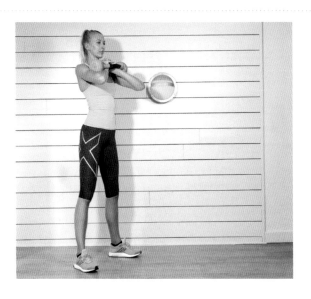

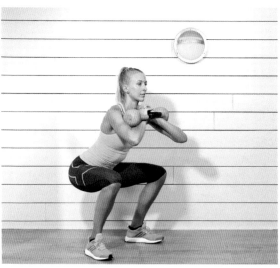

77

THE BOOTY-BUILDING BIBLE

I am on a constant mission to grow a bigger booty and as a result my favourite body part to train is glutes. I've spent my time as a personal trainer testing out all the best booty-building moves on myself and my clients and I am going to share them with you.

But before we go any further I need to tell you something: the key with glute training is to focus on the **mind–muscle connection**. Make sure that you're really thinking about using your glutes and giving them a good squeeze to avoid engaging surrounding muscles.

Got it? Let's go!

BACK EXTENSIONS

1. These can be done on a back extension machine or over a Swiss ball. Plant your feet and lean forwards to rest your tummy on the machine or ball, creating a straight line from your head to your toes.

2. Hinge forwards from the hips and drop your upper body towards the floor. On the way back up, pull from your hamstrings and glutes. Squeeze your booty at the top of the movement for a couple of seconds. Very slowly release. Repeat.

REVERSE LUNGE INTO KNEE RAISE

1. Stand with your feet hip-width apart. Take one leg behind you into a reverse lunge so both knees are at right-angles.

2. Stand back up by pushing through the front heel. As you do so, bring the back leg in front of you and lift the knee. Squeeze the opposite glute and push your hips forwards. Repeat. Complete all reps on one leg before switching to the other.

DONKEY KICKS

1. Kneel on the floor with your knees below your hips and arms below your shoulders.

2. Lift one leg, keeping it bent and your core engaged, until your hamstring is in line with your spine. Contract your glutes throughout this movement and hold the contraction at the top for a second, giving your glutes a good squeeze! Return your leg to the starting position and repeat. Once you have done all the reps on one leg, switch to the other.

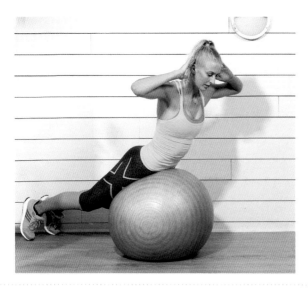

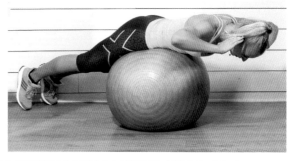

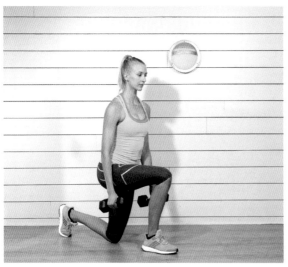

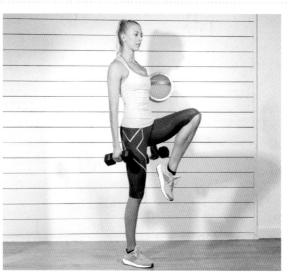

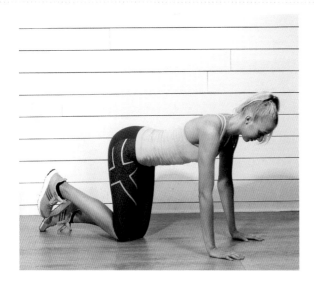

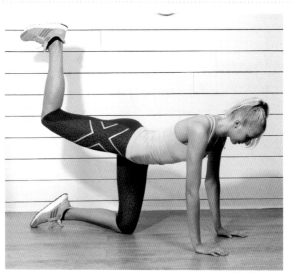

ELEVATED SINGLE-LEG GLUTE BRIDGE

1. Lie on the floor with a bench or block in front of you. Place one heel on the edge of the bench and relax the other leg.

2. Drive through the heel on the bench, extending your hips upwards and lifting your body off the ground. At the top of the movement, squeeze the glute of the leg on the bench for a second. Lower back down to the starting position, keeping tension on the glute and not resting back onto the floor completely before the next rep. Complete all reps on one leg before switching to the other.

As well as my personal favourites above, I need to give a shoutout to all the moves included earlier in the book that I absolutely love for booty building.

These include:

BARBELL HIP THRUSTS
see page 54

BARBELL SUMO DEADLIFTS
see page 54

BULGARIAN SPLIT SQUATS
see page 40

CURTSEY LUNGES
see page 58

BANDED GLUTE ACTIVATION WORK
see page 30

STEP-UPS
see page 42

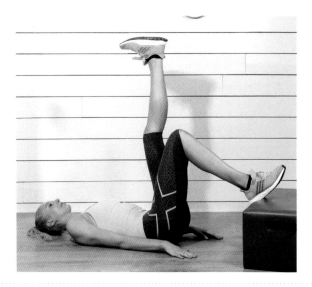
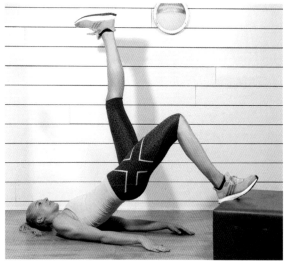

"Your mind will quit 100 times before your body ever does."

THE FORMIDABLE PULL-UP

By far the question I am most frequently asked is how to do a first pull-up or chin-up. These are super-challenging exercises which even the fittest people can struggle to execute as they require a lot of upper-body strength. However, that doesn't mean they're unachievable. There are two key things you need to do:

• General back and bicep training using the exercises outlined earlier in the book. This is necessary to build up muscle and strength in these areas.

• Pull-up-specific exercises on a regular basis. I recommend adding in a couple of these exercises once or twice a week to see rapid progression. Here are my top picks.

ECCENTRIC PULL-UPS

1. These are essential! Hold on to pull-up handles with your chosen grip. Using a step, jump up so you're holding your body off the floor with your chin just above the pull-up handles. Stabilise yourself.

2. Slowly, slowly, slowly release yourself down towards the floor, squeezing your back and biceps as you do so. Jump back up to the top and repeat.

Top tip: You can mix these up. Try doing 3 reps slowly, one super-duper-long slow rep or even 5 reps a little faster.

PULL-UP HOLDS

1. Hold on to pull-up handles with your chosen grip. Using a step, jump up so you're holding your body off the floor with your chin just above the pull-up handles. Stabilise yourself.

2. Lower yourself so that your arms are at a little less than a right-angle. Now hold. Stay here for as long as you can - count the seconds and try to increase your time! Once your arms extend to over a right-angle, lower yourself to the floor. Repeat until you can't do any more reps.

BANDED PULL-UPS

1. Place a large looped resistance band around the pull-up handles. Pop one of your knees into it. Grab the pull-up handles with your chosen grip and lift your feet off the floor.

2. From here use your upper body to pull yourself up so your chin passes the top of the bars. Then slowly lower back to the bottom, keeping your feet off the floor. Repeat until you can't do any more reps.

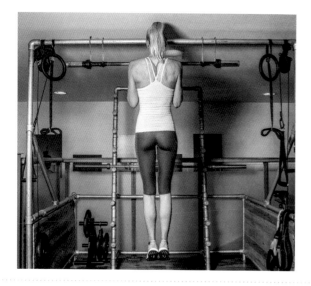

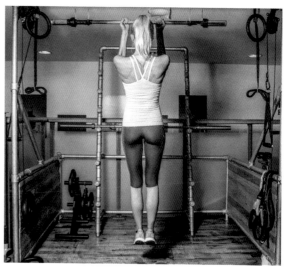

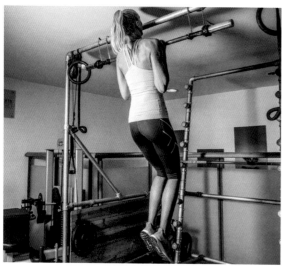

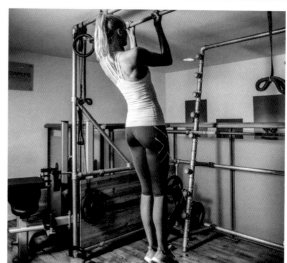

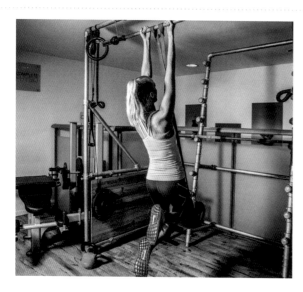

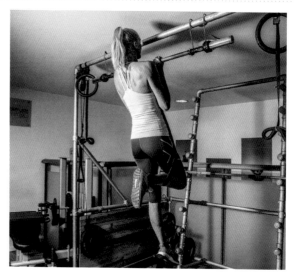

Top tip: Start with underhand-grip chin-ups. They are the easiest kind as they recruit more of your biceps. Then move to middle grip and wide grip as you get stronger. Remember too that you don't need to do loads of reps of these exercises. You can just do 3—4 sets of a few reps to get amazing results. Make sure you focus on time under tension and progression over time.

UNDERHAND:

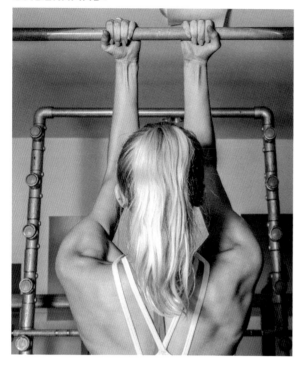

MIDDLE GRIP:

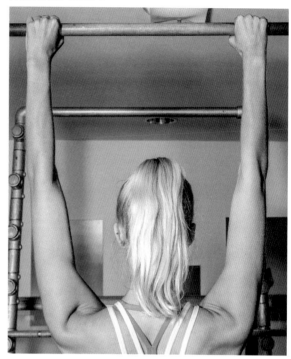

WIDE GRIP:

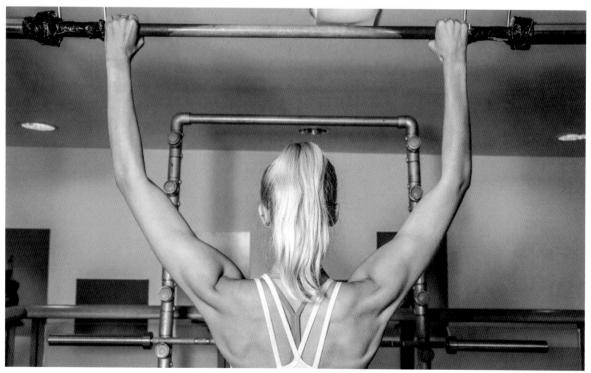

"Great things never came from comfort zones."

BUT WHAT ABOUT ABS?

Ahhh... abs. Everyone is obsessed with them, but are they really all that special? Having abs is not a direct reflection of how healthy you are. You can be super-strong, fit, happy and healthy with or without them. There is no use stressing yourself out because you haven't got them. It's much more important to focus on how you're performing in the gym and how you feel in your clothes than to fret over whether you have a defined stomach. You're so much more than that.

So, do you need to train them? Yes and no. You certainly don't need to be doing endless sets of crunches, sit-ups and twists. Instead, focus on engaging your abs during your weighted workouts and target them with a couple of key moves.

ENGAGING YOUR CORE

One of the awesome benefits of resistance training is that it uses your core in pretty much every single movement. However, many people are guilty of letting their core stability go when they are lifting, which increases the risk of injury. Don't let that be you! Ensure that you engage your core during every exercise. But how? Don't just 'suck in' your stomach. Instead imagine someone is about to punch you in the gut and brace your core for the impact.

TARGETING YOUR CORE

Training your core is essential in helping to stabilise your spine and support the rest of your training. However, contrary to popular belief, you don't need to train your abs every day. They need rest like any other muscle group. Instead I recommend doing a couple of isolation exercises one or two times per week at the end of your weighted workouts. Here are my top picks.

CORE

FOREARM PLANK

1. Come into a prone position on the floor, supporting your weight on your toes and forearms with your arms bent directly below your shoulders. Keep a straight line from your shoulders to your toes. Keep your core engaged. You can make this more challenging by adding in arm or leg lifts, toe taps or plate drags; the possibilities are endless!

TWISTING MOUNTAIN CLIMBERS WITH LEG LIFTS

1. Start in a plank position. Lift one leg off the floor and squeeze the glute.

2. Bring the leg down and under your body towards the opposite elbow, twisting your core slightly as you do so. Take the leg back into the lift, without returning it to the floor. Complete all reps on one leg before switching to the other side.

DEAD BUGS

1. These are my favourite and a slight variation on the traditional dead bug! Start by lying flat on the ground with your arms extended overhead.

2. Lift an arm and its opposite leg off the ground and reach the hand towards the toes, lifting your shoulder slightly off the floor and engaging your core. Release back to the floor. Repeat on the opposite side. That is one full rep.

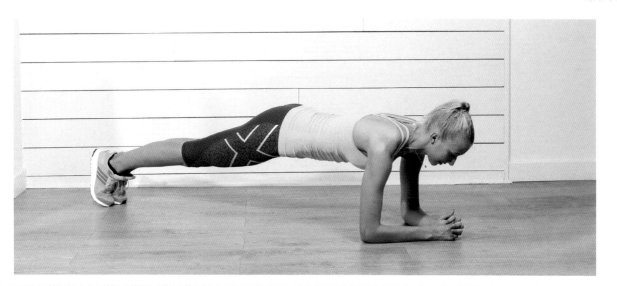

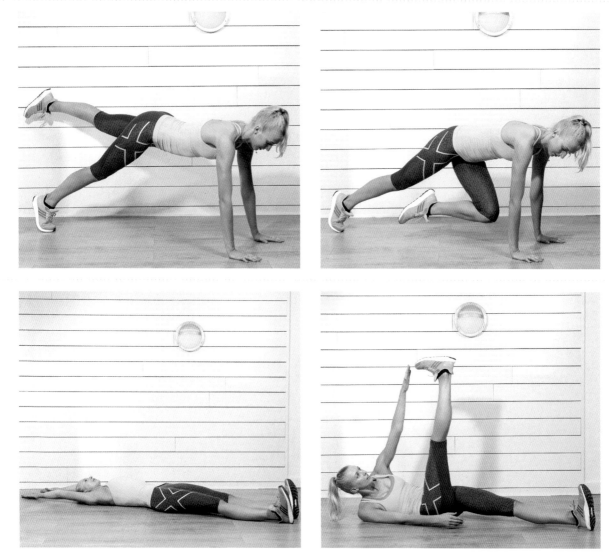

So that's it: my beginner's guide to lifting weights. I know it can seem overwhelming at first but I promise it gets easier over time. Once you start resistance training you will be hooked! I have done my best to cover the basic principles of resistance training, but there is only so much I can cram into this book and there will come a point when you want to know more. When that time comes I encourage you to get nerdy. Take things into your own hands. Read more books, do a course, look into research, ask an expert. This field is rapidly developing and there is always more to learn!

So what are you waiting for? Get your ass to the gym, try one of my workouts and work your way up from there. Soon you'll be a weight-lifting badass with a good ass to match!

"It never gets easier, you just get stronger."

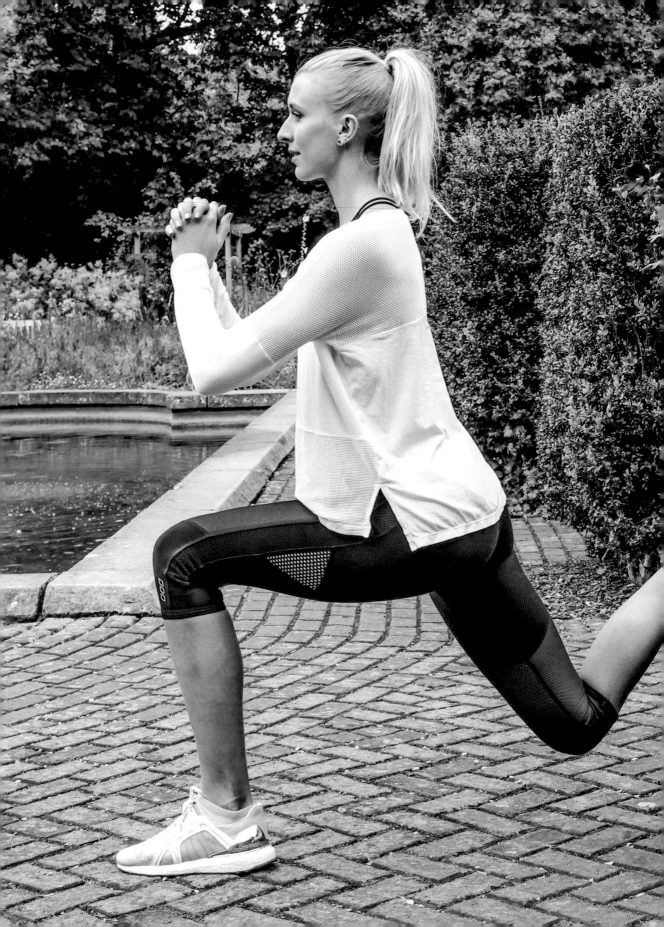

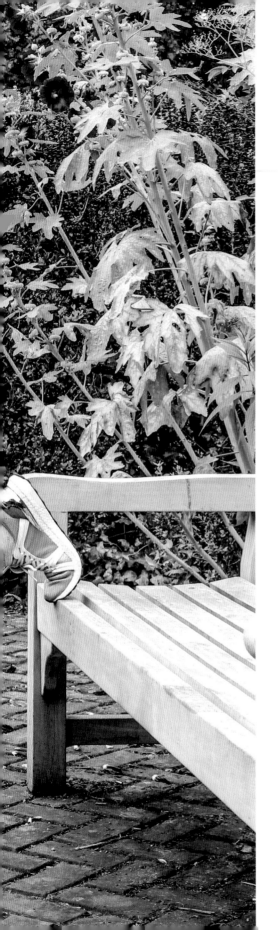

BODYWEIGHT HIIT TRAINING

Cardio is often demonised by dedicated weight lifters. They claim that it significantly inhibits the ability to develop muscle. Ignore these people. The impact of cardio on muscle building is small and you would have to be doing hours of the stuff for it to be a big issue. The benefits of cardio are huge, not only for your physical health but also for your mental health, and it shouldn't be shunned. Plus, it can be super-satisfying and fun!

You've probably heard about HIIT, or high-intensity interval training. It's all the rage right now and rightly so as it's a great form of exercise for busy people with minimal time. In a nutshell, it combines short periods of intense exercise with longer, less intense recovery periods (e.g., 20 seconds of exercise followed by 40 seconds of rest). This is an effective form of cardio which mobilises fat from adipose tissue stores, elevates your heart rate and increases blood circulation throughout your body. As a result you become fitter and faster and improve your heart health. I recommend this approach as it means that you can get a seriously sweaty cardio session done in a short time period. And the best part? These workouts require no equipment so can be completed anywhere, anytime.

WHAT YOU NEED:

- your bodyweight
- some wiggle room to jump about
- a timer — I recommend the app Seconds

THE WORKOUTS

There are endless ways in which you can structure your HIIT workouts and I can't even begin to cover them all. Instead I am going to show you my personal favourite method to smash out a quick 30-minute session. It's challenging, fun and effective. I like to use circuits of six to eight bodyweight exercises back to back. You do the first exercise for 30 seconds, then rest for 15 seconds, then move on to the second exercise for 30 seconds and so on.

You do this until you complete all of the exercises in the circuit, then rest for 60–90 seconds and do it all again – two, three or four times depending on the time available. I recommend mixing up lower-body, upper-body and full-body exercises to really get your blood pumping.

FULL BODY HIIT: BEGINNER

Remember to warm up before these workouts!

BURPEES

1. Stand with your feet hip-width apart. Drop your hands to the floor and kick your legs behind you so you're in a high plank position.

2. Jump your legs back in and stand back up, jumping into the air. You can raise your arms overhead to gain momentum. As you land back onto the floor, go straight into the next rep and repeat.

HIGH KNEES

1. Stand with your feet hip-width apart. Bring one knee up towards your chest, at waist height or higher.

2. Jump into the air and switch legs, bringing the other knee high and swinging your arms as you do so. Keep your chest upright throughout the movement and repeat.

JUMPING JACKS

1. Starting in a standing position with your hands by your sides and feet hip-width apart.

2. Jump your legs out to the sides while simultaneously lifting your arms overhead to form an X shape. Then jump back to the starting position. Stay light on your feet throughout the movement.

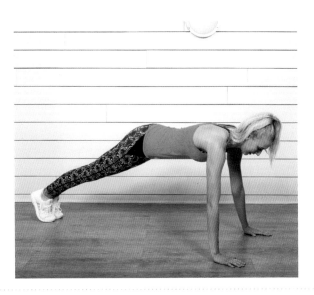
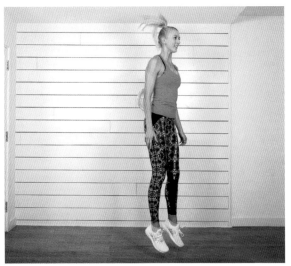
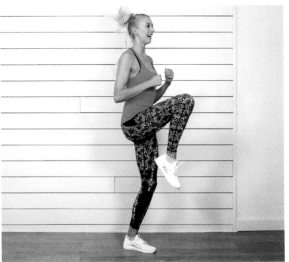
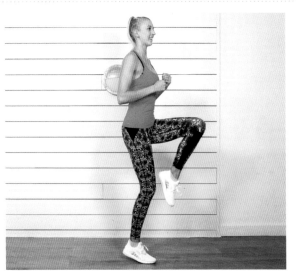
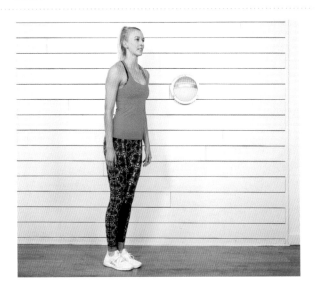
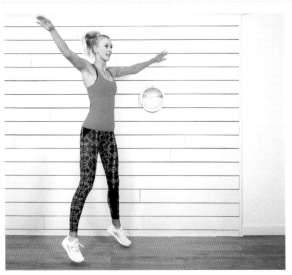

SQUAT WITH SIDE KICK

1. Stand with your feet hip-width apart. Lower yourself down into a squat position, keeping your torso upright.
2. Push up through your heels to return to standing. As you do so, kick one leg out to the side (hiii-YAH!). Then, as you lower your leg, go straight back into a squat. Repeat on the opposite side.

MOUNTAIN CLIMBERS

1. Go into a high plank position with your hands beneath your shoulders. Bend one leg and pull it forwards towards your elbow and then lower it back to the starting position.
2. Repeat with the opposite leg, keeping your core engaged and back straight. Now increase the speed!

PUSH-UPS

1. On the floor, come into a high plank position with your hands directly below your shoulders and feet together.
2. Bend your arms until your elbows are at a right-angle, lowering your chest towards the floor and keeping your core engaged and back straight. Straighten your arms to return to the starting position. If this is too challenging then this movement can be done on your knees. Just ensure there is a straight line from your head to your knees.

FOREARM PLANK

1. Come into a prone position on the floor, supporting your weight on your toes and forearms with your arms bent directly below your shoulders. Keep a straight line from your shoulders to your toes. Keep your core engaged.

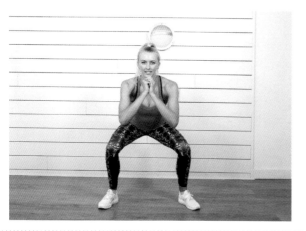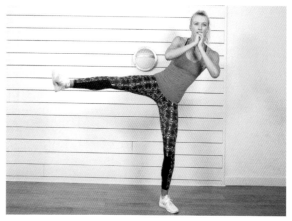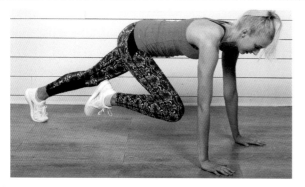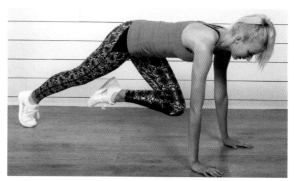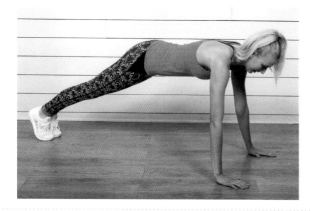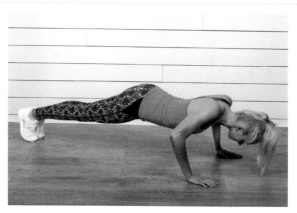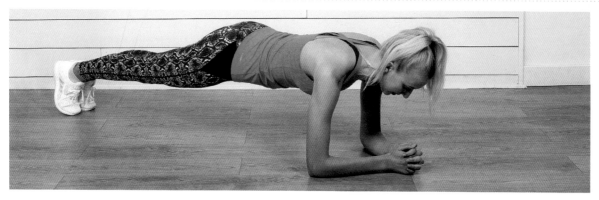

FULL BODY HIIT: ADVANCED

Remember to warm up before these workouts!

TUCK-JUMP BURPEES

1. Stand with your feet hip-width apart. Drop your hands to the floor and kick your legs behind you so you're in a high plank position.

2. Jump your legs back in and stand back up, jumping into the air and tucking your knees into your chest. As you land back onto the floor, go straight into the next rep and repeat.

COMMANDOS

1. Start in a low plank position on your toes and forearms. From here walk your hands up one at a time so your arms are extended and you're in a high plank position.

2. Gently, one arm at a time, lower yourself back down to a low plank position. The key is to keep your core stable throughout this whole movement. Minimal swaying is allowed!

JUMPING LUNGES

1. This is a toughie. Start standing with your feet hip-width apart. Jump up into the air and land in a lunge position with both legs bent at a right-angle.

2. Explode out of the movement and jump into the air, switching your legs as you do so. Land into a lunge on the opposite leg. Keep your torso upright throughout. Repeat.

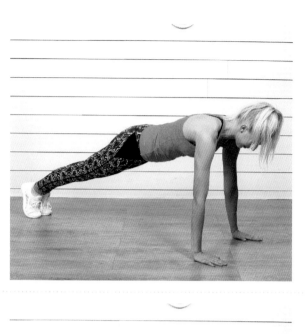

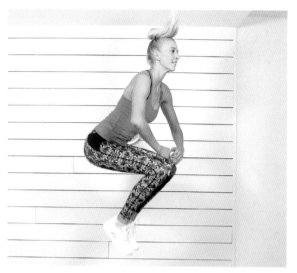

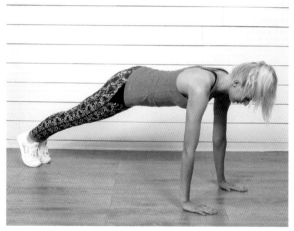

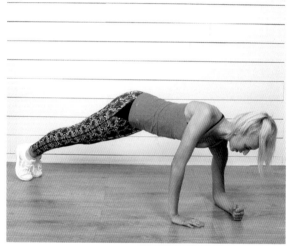

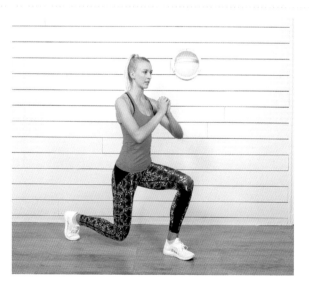

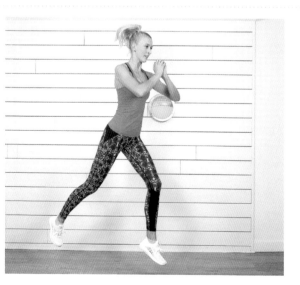

CRAB KICKS

1. Start in a seated position on the floor with your hands behind you and feet planted in front of you. Lift your body off the floor.

2. Kick one leg forwards and then explode up and lift both legs off the ground, switching sides in mid-air. Land softly with the opposite leg in the air. Repeat.

TUCK JUMPS

1. Start standing with your feet hip-width apart. Swing your arms and bend your legs slightly to get some momentum, jumping into the air as high as you can.

2. At the top of the movement, bring your knees high into your chest to perform a tuck movement. Then lower your legs to land – softly – in a standing position. Repeat.

PLANK JACKS

1. Come into a high plank position on the floor. Keep a straight line from your shoulders to your toes.

2. Jump your feet out to the sides as if you're doing a jumping jack, then jump back to the centre. Keep your core as stable as possible throughout this motion.

MOUNTAIN-CLIMBER PUSH-UPS

1. Go into a high plank position with your hands beneath your shoulders. Bend one leg and pull it forwards towards your elbow and lower it back to the starting position. Repeat with the opposite leg, keeping your core engaged and back straight.

2. After you have done this movement with both legs, drop down into a press up, lowering your chest towards the floor and bending your arms. Push back up to a plank position. That is one rep. Ouch!

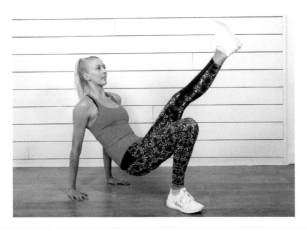 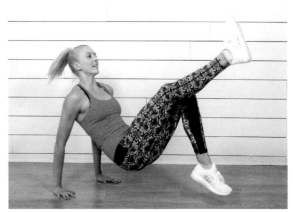

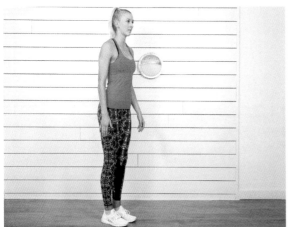 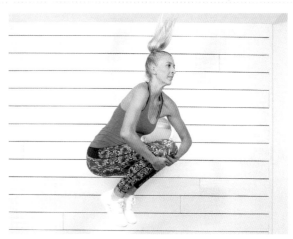

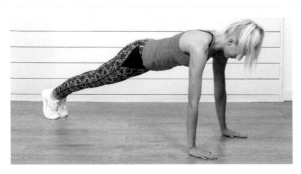 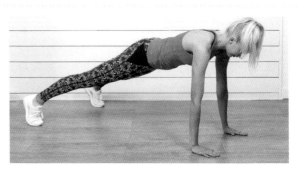

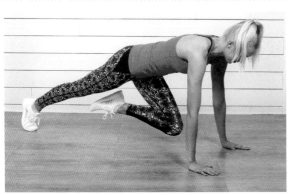 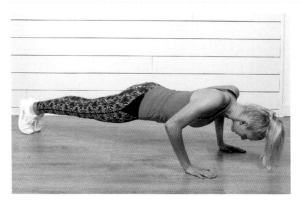

"You've got this."

HOW TO STEP IT UP

Once you've worked your way through these workouts, you may wonder where to go next. Here are a few simple tips for switching up your circuits and challenge yourself in new ways:

- **Change the exercises.**
Try adding in more challenging variations. For example, instead of doing a standard burpee, add a half twist or lateral jump to each rep!

- **Add more moves.**
Instead of doing six exercises go for seven or eight.

- **Increase the work time.**
Spend more time doing the exercises, for example 40 seconds instead of 30.

- **Reduce the rest time.**
Spend less time resting between the exercises, for example 10 seconds instead of 15.

- **Do more rounds.**
Complete the full circuit three or four times rather than twice.

- **Use equipment.**
If you're in a gym, don't be afraid to add in weighted exercises such as kettle bell swings, battle ropes, sledge pushes and so on.

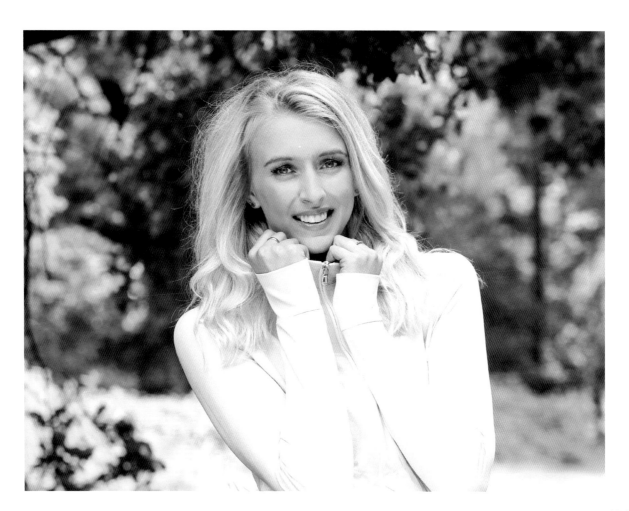

THE TABATA WORKOUTS

Tabata is a form of HIIT based around 4-minute workouts - perfect for when you're super-short on time. They consist of intervals of 20 seconds of work and 10 seconds of rest which are repeated eight times.

You can choose to do one to eight different exercises; however, I personally prefer two alternating exercises for simplicity's sake. I warn you now, these may be short but they're certainly not sweet!

SIX EXAMPLE TABATA WORKOUTS

BEGINNER	INTERMEDIATE	ADVANCED
High knees and bodyweight squats	Squat jumps and jumping jacks	Crab kicks and tuck–jump burpees
Mountain climbers and alternating bodyweight reverse lunges	Push–ups and squats with side kick	Commandos and jumping lunges

HOW TO USE THESE WORKOUTS

As I said before, not only do we need to lift weights to get stronger but we also need to get moving to get fitter and faster. HIIT is a quick and effective way to squeeze in cardiovascular training, get a sweat on and improve your fitness levels.

So, when should you do these workouts? The answer is whenever you can. You can fit these into your schedule as you please, for example doing some circuits as a stand-alone workout or adding a quick tabata session onto the end of a weights session. And you can pretty much do them as often as you like! This is **your** training regime so do what **you** enjoy and what fits into **your** life. My only advice is to avoid doing HIIT every single day, as it is very high impact and can be extremely taxing on your body and central nervous system, and to avoid doing it at the expense of weight training. Ensure you keep a balance of both cardio and resistance training to reap the most benefits. Oh, and don't forget: once these workouts get easy, switch them up! Your body needs to be challenged to be changed.

THE SKIPPING ROPE WORKOUTS

Skipping is highly underrated. It is an amazing way to squeeze in a high-intensity cardio workout with minimal equipment. Try out these two workouts when you're short on time.

10-MINUTE SKIPPING WORKOUT

1 minute normal pace

1 minute high knees

1 minute normal pace

1 minute as fast as you can

Rest 1 minute

1 minute normal pace

1 minute single leg (right)

1 minute single leg (left)

1 minute normal pace

1 minute as fast as you can

15-MINUTE AMRAP

100 normal skips

50 skips high knees

10 burpees

30 second plank

AMRAP stands for 'as many rounds as possible'. Basically this means that you try to complete a series of exercises in sequence as many times as you can within the set time period (e.g. 15 minutes), taking a rest when you need it. These are a great way to track progress as week by week you will be able to complete more rounds!

THIS IS JUST THE BEGINNING...

I have covered the key areas of resistance training and bodyweight HIIT training, as they are two forms of exercise which really do help you to achieve a strong, lean and fit body. However, there are **so** many other ways to work out. Nowadays there is something for everyone, from classes such as body pump, boxing and barre through to sports such as swimming, rock climbing and tennis. You can even do Beyoncé dance classes! I will eat my hat if you can't find a form of exercise which you enjoy! So don't be afraid to experiment and try new things, and, if it makes it easier, rope a friend in for the ride.

Top tip: If you're doing a session which combines cardio and weights, ensure that the cardio is at the end. If you do it prior to lifting, you will tire the muscles, which can sacrifice good form and increase the risk of injury.

FORMULATING YOUR ROUTINE

You're probably feeling slightly overwhelmed by the sheer volume of information you have received from this book already. Don't worry, I get it. To help make all of this a little more digestible and practical, let's talk about how to use this knowledge to formulate a personalised routine for you.

Your exercise regime should always be challenging you and, as a result, your fitness levels and physique should always be progressing. Step out of your comfort zone. Lift heavier weights. Run a little faster or walk a little further. The moments when you feel like giving up are the ones when the most changes are made. Keep pushing and I promise it will be worth it.

So, the three main things you need to focus on including are:

- resistance training
- cardiovascular training
- enjoyment!

HOW OFTEN SHOULD I TRAIN?

The choice is yours. Evaluate your schedule and find times when you can slot in a cheeky workout. Be realistic with this. Don't set yourself up for failure by planning to train six days a week when you're an extremely busy bee. In reality, you don't need to go to the gym every day or for hours at a time. A great place to start is with two or three short, sharp and effective workouts per week and go from there.

HOW SHOULD I TRAIN?

If you can't tell by now, I am a pretty big fan of resistance training and I recommend that everyone tries to incorporate it into their fitness routine in some capacity. As someone who has had their life and body transformed by this way of training, I highly recommend you give it a go. Why not start out with one or two weighted workouts per week? However, exercising in any form is amazing and a positive step forwards for your health. Try out a mixture of weighted workouts, cardiovascular training, classes, walking and anything else you fancy. Just focus on pushing your body and getting sweaty in an enjoyable way. The HIIT workouts earlier in this book are great if you're short on time, but don't limit yourself to these. Try a park bootcamp, go for a run or hop into a local spinning class. The possibilities are endless!

WHAT FORM OF CARDIO SHOULD I DO?

In this book I have focused on HIIT cardio as it is quick and effective, meaning you can squeeze it into almost any schedule. However, this isn't the only approach. Low-intensity steady-state cardio, or LISS, such as jogging and cycling, is also effective. The long and short of it is that HIIT is more stressful on the body but more time efficient. LISS is more time-consuming but more gentle on the body. There is nothing wrong with doing a combination of both, alternating them or combining them. The amazing thing about cardio is that it can be integrated into your life in so many ways! You can use it to transport you to work (e.g., cycling or walking) or to explore your surroundings (during activities such as hiking). This all counts as exercise! Pick your poison: it is a case of personal preference and what fits in with your schedule.

ARE THERE ANY DAILY ACTIVITIES I CAN DO?

Yes! To make positive changes in your overall health it is vital to increase your daily activity level, and I don't just mean squats and running. I'm talking about walking, the most undervalued way to get active. I walk everywhere I can and it's an absolute game changer. Sure, it isn't a high-intensity form of exercise but the benefits are huge. It gets you moving and, if you go outdoors, it gives you some much needed fresh air. Walking also has psychological benefits as it gives you time to reflect and mull over your thoughts, plans and ideas. I always find that when I am walking my stress levels reduce and my mind clears, making the rest of my day more productive

and efficient. In modern society, where we spend so much time sat down at work and at home, walking more is an essential but simple step to better health.

IS THERE ANYTHING I SHOULD AVOID?

Try not to train the same muscles on two consecutive days e.g. training legs on Monday and Tuesday. Not only will this make it challenging for you to train as effectively but it actually makes it harder for your muscles to recover, grow and repair.

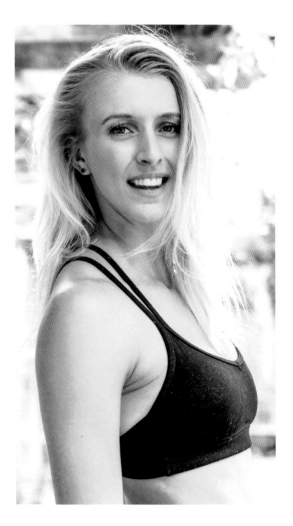

EXAMPLE WORKOUT ROUTINES

	MON	TUES	WEDS
BEGINNER	Full-body weights	Rest	Jog around the park
INTERMEDIATE	Lower-body weights	Spinning class	Upper-body weights
ADVANCED	Lower-body weights	Upper-body weights	Home HIIT workout

Note: These workout routines are **examples** and are **not** prescriptive. I have kept the weekends free as most people like to relax on these days. However, you can train on Saturday and/or Sunday if you want.

MY EXAMPLE WORKOUT ROUTINE

As someone who loves lifting weights, I aim to do 3–4 resistance training sessions a week. I take 1–2 rest days (or more if needed) and like to incorporate some sweaty cardio too.

	MON	TUES	WEDS
EXAMPLE	Lower-body weights	Home HIIT workout	Upper-body weights

THURS	FRI	SAT	SUN
Rest	Gym class	Rest	Rest
Rest	Home HIIT workout	Rest	Rest
Full-body weights	Jog around the park	Rest	Rest

THURS	FRI	SAT	SUN
Rest	Legs	Boxing class	Rest (with a long walk)

RECOVERY

Now, let's talk about perhaps the most important element of your fitness routine: recovery. How well you facilitate your recovery from exercise will drastically impact the speed at which you progress and the results you will achieve. If you take the time to look after yourself on every step of your fitness journey, I promise the road to a stronger, fitter and healthier you will be much smoother.

I encourage you to focus on the three S's: sleep, stress and stretching.

SLEEP

As our lives get busier and busier, something has to give, and that something is often sleep. Staying up late, working into the early hours and coming in the next day running on empty has become something people brag about. In reality, no one should be showing off about a lack of sleep - especially at work, as it directly affects your performance.

Sleep is undervalued. This is when your brain and body grow and repair. Sleep helps your muscles to strengthen and develop, it plays an important role in regulating your metabolism and immune system, and it facilitates learning and memory function. The more sleep you get, the better you function - not just physically with increased energy levels but also mentally with improved concentration and productivity. Sleep also helps you to have the right mindset to keep your motivation levels high so that you make healthy choices.

How much of this magic stuff do you need? The general consensus is around 8 hours per night. Here are my top tips for clocking up those valuable Zzzs:

• Create a night-time routine. Try to have a series of activities which you do before bed and which cue your body that it's time for sleep - for example, washing your face, brushing your teeth and reading a few pages of a book.

• On a similar note, try to go to sleep at the same time each night to help your body clock get used to a regular schedule.

• Turn out the lights, and not just the ones on the ceiling! Our bodies release a hormone called melatonin when it's dark, and this helps to make us sleepy. So switch off your lamps when it gets late and reduce the brightness of your screens. Even better, try to avoid screen time at all for the final hour before sleep.

• While we're talking about light, invest in some heavy curtains or black-out blinds to keep your room as dark as possible to help facilitate a good night's sleep.

• Put down the coffee. We all know this by now but caffeine and sleep don't get along. So try to avoid having caffeine-loaded drinks in the afternoon or evening.

• Put down the water too. Try not to drink huge quantities of any liquids close to bed time, as you may end up waking in the night to go for a wee.

• Write it down. Often when we get into bed our minds start racing and we can't get thoughts out of our head. I find that having a small notepad and pen next to my bed helps as I can just note down anything that comes to mind. This helps to clear my thoughts so I can sleep peacefully.

• Prepare for the next day. I find that writing a to-do list for the next day, prepping my meals and snacks, and laying out my clothes really helps me to sleep well. It assures me that I will wake up and be able to start my day on the right foot.

• Take a nap. They aren't just for when you're hungover. They can actually be super-useful if you're having a dip in your energy levels. Just try to keep them short and sweet (under an hour) and don't have one close to bed time.

• Work out. I find that when I exercise it is so much easier to fall asleep as my body is tired. So get moving and use up your energy!

STRESS

Stress is almost unavoidable nowadays and I have certainly fallen victim to it (and still do!). We've all felt it in some form or another, with one of the most common sources being work. With many jobs involving high-pressure situations, ever-rising targets and looming deadlines, it's no wonder we're feeling overwhelmed. What many people don't know is that stress leads to the release of a hormone called cortisol. This can be useful in small doses. However, if it is chronically elevated, it can actually have negative impacts on your body, mind and overall health. Chronic stress has been linked to fatigue, muscle tension, poor sleep, high blood pressure, anxiety and irritability. Furthermore, it can affect your energy levels and how well you recover from exercise. Basically, stress is bad news and I am here to share my top tips to combat it:

• First things first, identify what is causing your stress, whether it's your home life, your workload or anything in between. Simply identifying what's causing it can immediately make you feel more in control of your emotions.

• Disconnect. Technology is a constant cause of stress, and even once we leave the office we can't escape the ping of our email notifications. Start by turning your phone to airplane mode or completely off for half an hour and work your way up from there.

• Use your commute. Your journey to work doesn't have to be stressful. Use it as a chance to relax and listen to some educational or inspirational podcasts such as TED Talks Radio. This means you can start and end your working day on a positive note.

• Take time off. If you're a workaholic like me, you might struggle with the concept of days off. However, giving yourself time to switch off from business actually allows you to think more clearly and work more efficiently when you get back to it. Plus it gives you an opportunity to spend time with your loved ones or have some solo down time.

PSST! While we're talking about resting, let's touch on rest days. It is a common misconception that the quickest way to get fit is to train all day every day. What if I told you it's better to do less? I recommend taking at least one if not two rest days each week to support muscle growth and recovery between your workouts.

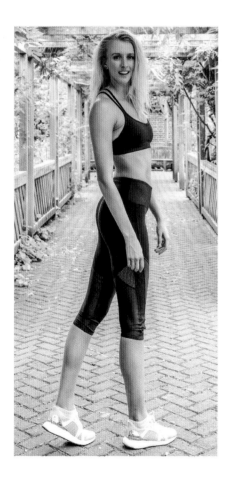

• When you have time off, put on an out-of-office email alert to avoid the stress of feeling like you have to reply immediately.

• Say no! I have learned the hard way that if you take on too many projects, you can become overwhelmed and find that you don't do anything effectively. Instead, don't be afraid to politely decline projects which are not worth your time. Do less, but better.

• Talk it out. You know what they say: a problem shared is a problem halved. Talk through what's bothering you with your friends, family or partner. It is useful to get an outsider's opinion as they often see things from a different perspective to you.

• Find some activities which relax you and allow your mind to disconnect from your worries. This could be anything from filling out a colouring book (my personal favourite!) to calling a friend or popping on a face mask. Identify what relaxes you and schedule it into your life. Whether it's for 10 minutes a day or an hour a week, just do something for yourself.

• Get moving. You've heard it before: exercise reduces stress and releases endorphins – chemicals which lead to positive and happy feelings. So get a sweat on and smile :-)

• On the subject of exercise, boxing is a fantastic stress reliever. There is nothing more empowering than smashing the living daylights out of a bag. Trust me!

• Surround yourself with positive people. Identify your true loved ones – the people who make you happy, empower you and genuinely want what's best for you. Prioritise these people and spend time with them. Their positive vibes will rub off on you!

STRETCHING

Everyone is guilty of doing exercise and then forgetting to stretch out afterwards – at least I certainly am! Post-workout stretching and regular foam rolling are undervalued and often neglected, when in fact they are essential. Let me explain.

You might have heard gym-goers talking about their 'DOMS' and wondered what on earth they were on about. DOMS stands for delayed-onset muscle soreness and refers to the aches you feel in your muscles in the days following a tough workout. Supporting recovery through stretching, foam rolling, adequate sleep, reduced stress and good nutrition can help to reduce this soreness.

Stretching out your muscles can lead to improved flexibility, range of motion and posture. It also increases blood flow and nutrient supply to your muscles and reduces the risk of injury. Basically, the benefits are huge, so don't avoid it! I share my top stretching tips on page 32.

Foam rolling is another name for self-myofascial release, a self-massage technique used to release muscular tightness and trigger points. It uses deep compression to relax tight muscles and break up adhesions formed between muscle layers and their surroundings. This helps to ensure your muscles maintain flexibility, allows normal blood flow to return and encourages the restoration of healthy tissue. Plus it helps to avoid build-up of tension and knots and subsequent discomfort or pain.

So how do you do it? Apply moderate pressure to a specific muscle or muscle group using the roller and your bodyweight. Roll slowly, no more than an inch per second. Once you find a tight area, pause and try to relax the muscles. You should start to feel the tension releasing and the discomfort lessening. If an area is too painful for you to apply direct pressure, try rolling the surrounding area and gradually work up to the trigger point. The goal is to ensure your muscles are healthy – this isn't a challenge to cause as much pain as possible! Once the tension has lessened in an area, move on to the next spot.

Start out with a softer, smooth foam roller and move on to more firm ones with different textures to help ease out any deeper tension. Try not to foam roll your lower back. Instead use a tennis ball to target that area. If you have neck pain, consult a physio as this area is more sensitive.

HOW OFTEN SHOULD I STRETCH AND FOAM ROLL? AND WHEN?

I recommend that you use dynamic stretching before and static stretching after **every single workout**. Aim to do 5-10 minutes as an absolute minimum!

Foam rolling is extremely beneficial pre-workout and pre-stretching to increase circulation to your muscles. However, it can seem like a lot to foam roll, stretch and work out all at once! So I like to do foam rolling at a separate time. I aim to do it two or three times a week for about 15-30 minutes. I do it in the comfort of my own home (foam rollers are super-cheap) while I watch a documentary or listen to a podcast. Multi-tasking at its finest!

PROGRESS

Now it comes down to the nitty gritty, the results. By taking a balanced approach to training which combines resistance training with moving more, getting a sweat on and having fun, you **will** lean down, tone up and drop inches. However, let's be real here. This approach will not make you have a six-pack in 6 days or drop 10 pounds in a week. That's not the goal. Those results are unsustainable and unenjoyable. I guarantee that to achieve them you would be slaving away for hours in the gym and depriving yourself of valuable nutrients. By taking a balanced approach you are saying no to yo-yo dieting and short-term success. Instead you will feel amazing, energised and happy and you will get fitter, stronger and faster. You will simultaneously lose weight and gain a glow, and these results will last long into the future.

Tracking progress is essential. It shows you how far you've come and is a constant source of motivation. Here are my top five things to track to check how you're doing:

- **Your scale weight.**
Now, this should be taken with a **hefty** pinch of salt, especially as you will be doing resistance training. As you simultaneously gain muscle and lose fat, the scales may not move but your body can **completely** transform. There is a significant difference between weight loss and fat loss. Muscle is more dense than fat so, although you may not lose weight, you will be losing inches, toning up and looking leaner. So, alongside the scales, I recommend using...

- **Pictures and measurements.**
Take pictures of yourself in the same undies or bikini from the front, back and side as well as measurements of your hips, bust and waist. Then retake these every week, fortnight or month and collate them all in a document or table so you can easily see your progression.

- **How your clothes fit.**
The scale may not be moving but your clothes could fit totally differently. Try on your favourite pair of jeans and see how they fit on your booty, hips and waist.

- **Your overall appearance.**
Take a look at your skin, hair and nails. I promise that by training hard, eating well and nourishing your body these will radically improve and you will glow from the inside out!

- **How you feel.**
You can progress in so many more ways than how you look, so it is super-important to consider how you feel and function. Look at how you're performing in the gym. Are you feeling strong and energised? Are you progressing? How well are you recovering from your sessions? Don't forget to check your mindset too. Are you motivated, happy and feeling positive? These are all valuable indicators of your progress.

GOAL SETTING

Setting goals is an essential part of any health and fitness journey. Carefully selected goals can help to keep you motivated and on track. As part of a balanced approach, I recommend setting ones which aren't just based on your appearance. Sure, you can aim to lose 5 pounds, drop a dress size or fit into your old jeans, but it is important to focus on your health too. Try aiming to do your first pull-up or run your first 5 km. This encourages you to see beyond how you look and into how you feel, how you function and how fit and healthy you really are.

Here are my top tips for setting fitness goals:

• Keep them SMART - that is: specific, measurable, achievable, realistic and time managed.

• Only set a couple of goals to begin with, so you can focus your time and energy on them. Too many may be overwhelming.

• Keep the goals small at first and work up to more challenging ones - you're changing your life after all! Plus, setting small goals means you're more likely to succeed in the beginning, which keeps you motivated.

• Write them down and return to them on a regular basis to evaluate your progress.

• Make them public. Stick them on your wall so you see them every day and tell your friends and family so they can support your efforts.

• Don't feel the pressure to set aesthetic goals just because everyone else is. Try to include at least one goal which isn't based directly on your appearance, for example training 3 days a week, drinking 2 litres of water a day or going for a morning walk.

• Focus on inclusion not exclusion, especially with food. Try to avoid saying you can't have 'bad food' and instead just focus on including more of the good stuff. This helps to maintain a positive relationship with food.

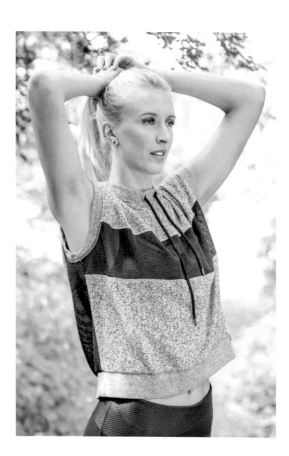

BUT... I CAN'T FIT TRAINING INTO MY DAY!

Yes you can! It is a case of prioritisation and working out how fitness can fit into **your** life. Everyone has different schedules, roles and responsibilities. There is someone out there busier than you that is fitting in their workouts, so you can too! I find the easiest way to facilitate a healthy lifestyle is to organise your days in such a way that exercise becomes part of your routine. There are a whole host of ways you can do this...

BECOME A MORNING PERSON

I personally find it so much easier to train first thing in the morning before I make up an excuse. If I train in the evening, I find that by 5 pm I have come up with something better to do... like watch cat videos on YouTube. If you smash your training session early doors, you're less likely to back out of it. There's no better feeling than getting it done before work and starting your day on the right foot. However, I understand that not everyone loves mornings as much as me, and trust me I never used to either. I made myself into a morning person and I have a few tricks up my sleeve to help you do the same.

TOP TIPS TO BECOME A MORNING PERSON

• Get to bed an hour earlier if you're going to wake an hour earlier. Lack of sleep isn't cool and means you'll have less energy to power through your morning workout.

• Put your alarm clock on the other side of the room so that you have to get out of bed to turn it off.

• Once you're out of bed, brush your teeth and drink a glass of water. These activities really wake you up and make it harder to return to your duvet!

• Plan ahead. Schedule in your workout, lay out your clothes and plan your journey if you're leaving the house. This means you'll have fewer opportunities to make excuses the next day.

• Book in to an early-morning gym class. The late cancellation charge will make you get out of bed!

• Think positively. You can see early mornings as a living hell or as a chance to get ahead of the game and work towards your goals. The power is in your hands to change your mindset and choose the latter.

• Stick with it. I promise that after a couple of weeks of early rises your body clock will start to adapt and it will become easier and easier, and perhaps even enjoyable!

If your schedule simply doesn't allow morning workouts, just squeeze your workouts in whenever you can, morning, noon or night. There is no perfect time to train. It doesn't matter as long as it gets done!

MAKE A SCHEDULE

My life is one big schedule; I have to-do lists, timetables, spreadsheets and wall calendars coming out of my ears! This level of scheduling might be daunting for some people, but I do recommend that everyone tries to incorporate the basics, such as diaries and to-do lists, into their lives. Here's my personal way that I schedule in my weekly workouts:

• To start off I have a diary. I use a paper one as I am traditional and there's nothing better than scribbling things out! (However, the one on your phone will do.) I like to use a 'page per day' diary to give me plenty of room for writing. In here I write all my plans as soon as I make them, including the exact timings, locations, and so on.

• On a weekend I will look ahead to my diary for the following week and assess the situation. This is when I will work out exactly what days and times I will be working out. I will add these into the diary and book in any classes that I need to do in advance. Additionally, I will take note of any days when I will struggle to get healthy food or be on the go, and plan in meal-prepping for those days.

• Each afternoon or evening I will plan the next day in more detail. I will look through my diary and write a note on my phone of my full schedule. This will include details such as when I wake up, what workout I will be doing, key tasks I need to complete and any journey times I need to factor in, all in chronological order (see example on the following page).

• As the day goes on, I delete items and tasks from my list. The ultimate satisfaction!

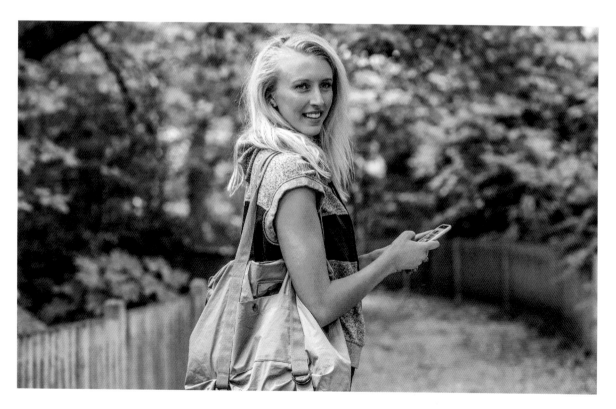

Example to-do list for a day

Get up at 6am

Leave house 6.30am

Train 6.45—7.45am at gym

Home 8am

Shower, breakfast and
ready by 9am

MORNING TASKS:
write 500 words for book

send follow-up emails to
Activewear stockists

edit one YouTube video
and make thumbnail

12.30pm lunch at home

Leave 1pm

2pm meeting at Headline:
SW3 4RF

Leave 3pm

4pm meeting at Active in
Style: SW4 6TH

Leave 5pm

Grab dinner on the go:
local Pret

6.30pm host panel event at
Grace Belgravia: SW1 8JK

TOP TIPS FOR A DAILY TO-DO LIST

• Include specific timings – for example, when you wake up, what time you need to be at each appointment. I also find including 'leaving times' important so that meetings don't overrun and I'm less likely to be late.

• Factor in any travel times and include locations (e.g., postcodes) to be easily entered into a journey planner app or sat nav.

• Use a buffer system. We often underestimate how long tasks and journeys take. So give yourself some leeway by adding on an extra bit of time for each activity. You never know what might crop up and throw you off schedule. This also puts you under less time pressure and reduces stress levels.

• Try to set yourself a maximum of three main tasks to do in a set time period to avoid feeling overwhelmed and unsatisfied if you can't complete everything. I recommend ordering these from most important to least important and trying to complete the hardest task first, to get it out of the way.

• Focus on one task at a time. Multi-tasking is a nightmare and often leads to inefficiency. To improve your productivity, focus on one task at a time and give it all your effort. This include your workouts – turn your phone onto airplane mode and leave the emails and calls for later.

• Factor in meals and workouts. Schedule in your workout including post-workout refuelling, showering, and so on. For meals, try to plan what you could eat, what options are available to you and whether you can prepare something to take on the go.

MAKE IT EASY FOR YOURSELF

We humans have a knack for making up excuses and we can find almost any reason to avoid exercising and eating well. Which is exactly why we need to find ways to make it easier for ourselves to live a healthy lifestyle. Try these top tips:

• If you're doing gym-based workouts, try to sign up to a gym that's easily accessible. It's much harder to motivate yourself to drive 40 minutes to the gym than to walk to one 15 minutes away. If that's a challenge in itself, just squeeze in a home workout!

• Keep your sessions short. It's more achievable to fit in a 30- or 40-minute workout than a 2-hour one!

• Remove temptation. I can't have cashew butter in my house, because I will eat the whole jar! Recognise your weaknesses and remove them from your vicinity. If you live with others and can't get rid of foods you find tempting, at least try to make them less accessible by putting them in hard-to-reach places. This gives you more time to think about what you're doing before you delve into a packet of biscuits.

• Facilitate healthy eating. Make nutritious food easily accessible. Have pre-cut carrot sticks in the fridge and keep a fruit bowl on the table. Also, organise your food storage. In the fridge divide up your fresh produce. For example, you could have a shelf for protein, one for fruit, one for veg, one for carbs and one for fats (e.g. cheese and eggs). This allows you to easily navigate the fridge to find exactly what you want. The same goes with your store cupboards. Keep your healthy ingredients (such as beans, chopped tomatoes, oats and rice) in easy reach. Keep the chocolate and treats on the top shelf and out of direct eyesight.

• Bulk up. By that I mean make things in bulk. If you're cooking a Bolognese, double up the portion, or if you're baking a chicken breast shove another one in the oven. Whatever excess you make, pop it in a container and keep it in the fridge. This gives you healthy food which you can access quickly and easily.

• Keep healthy snacks (such as fruit, nuts or homemade snack bars) in your bag. This gives you less of an excuse to buy that bar of Dairy Milk you're eyeing up.

• Keep yourself motivated. Remind yourself why you're doing this. Write it down on a piece of paper, stick it somewhere unavoidable and read it every day. Use social media to your advantage and follow inspiring fitness accounts. Make an epic pre-workout playlist you put on to get you pumped. Tell your friends about your goals so that they can hold you accountable or even join you on your fitness journey.

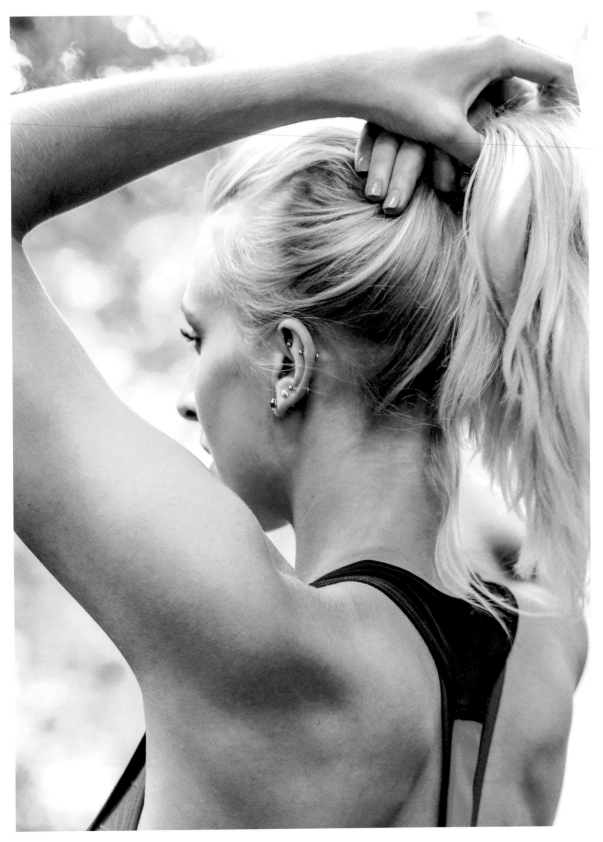

USE YOUR TIME WISELY

Be honest with yourself. How much time do you spend on activities such as watching TV, scrolling through Instagram or browsing online shops? Wouldn't this be much better spent challenging yourself in the gym or nourishing yourself by cooking a homemade meal? It is amazing how much more time we have to work towards our fitness goals when we simply switch time-wasting activities for more productive ones. However, that isn't to say that you can never watch trashy TV, but maybe try multi-tasking by stretching, foam rolling or even squat jumping while you do it!

BE REALISTIC

So you have your own business to run, three kids to raise or a hectic social life. That's okay. Be aware of this, accept it and work around it. You may not be able to train as much as you want, but make sure that the sessions you get in count. You may not be able to cook fresh meals every day, but make sure that your food choices are balanced. Don't be hard on yourself. It is not about being perfect. It is about doing the best you can and making small changes which will benefit your long-term health and happiness.

FIND YOUR BALANCE

Exercise **can** be enjoyable and **can** be incorporated into your life in a fun and sustainable way. It is a learning curve. You need to find a balance between sweaty workouts and your social life, between strength training and cardio, between pushing your body and giving it rest. This balance is completely personal to you, your body and your preferences. Don't be afraid to forge your own path and find a specific approach that works for you whether that's entering triathlons or dancing around your bedroom. Sustainability is key so if you can stick with it, then sod what anyone else thinks!

Time for a reality check...

We're coming to the end of the Move section of the book, and I admit there's a lot to take in and it can be hard to know where to start. Don't panic. Just focus on setting yourself a couple of small goals such as eating a healthy breakfast every day and doing two workouts a week, then work from there. You are *changing your life*. That's a pretty big deal.

You will have to put in the work to achieve your goals. I can promise you that it will get easier over time. Soon the things which seem like a chore now will become a habit and the challenges will become easy. You just need to stick with it and trust the process. The power is in your hands. Use it.

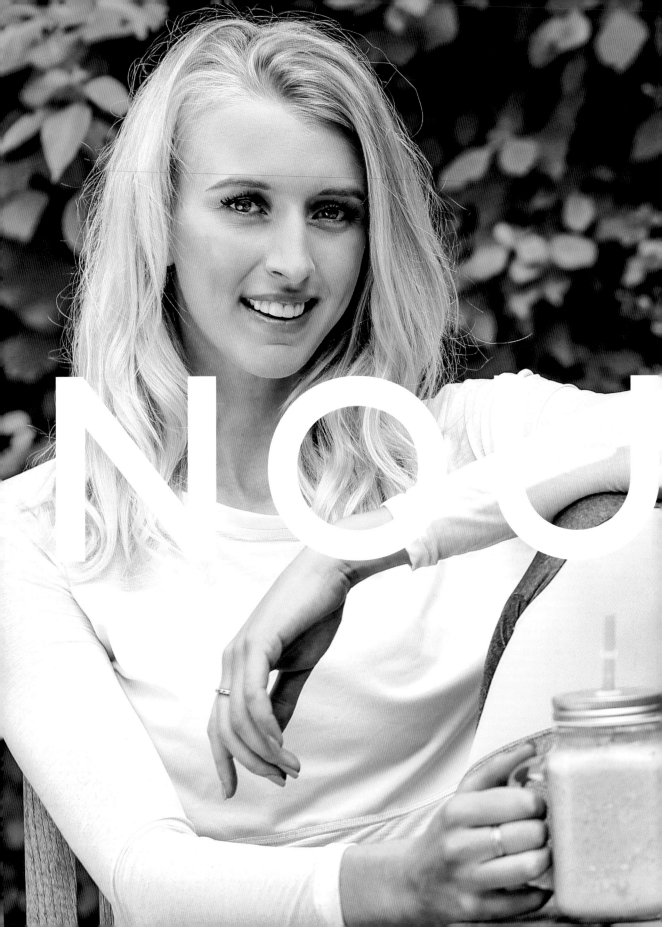

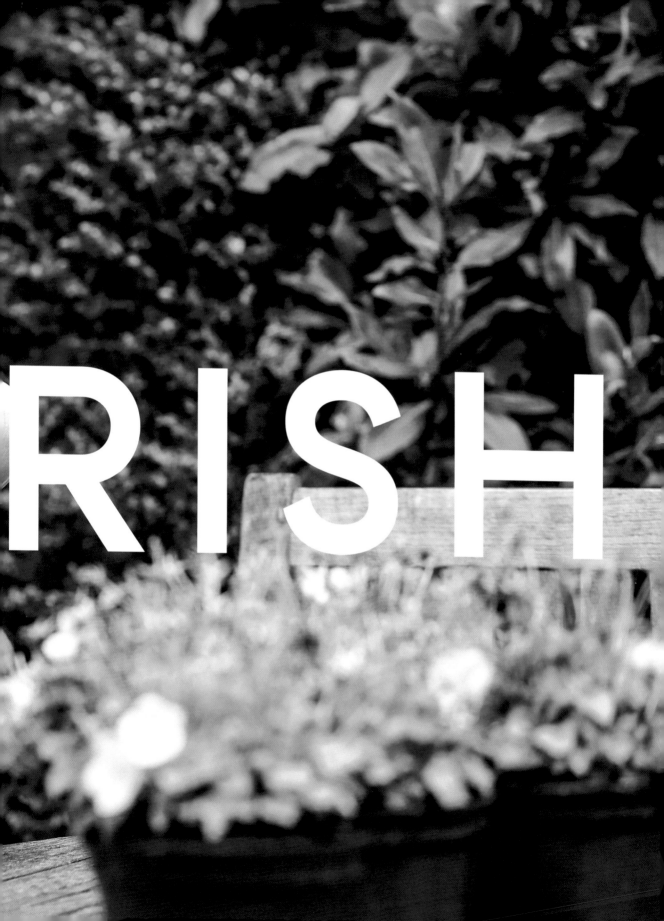

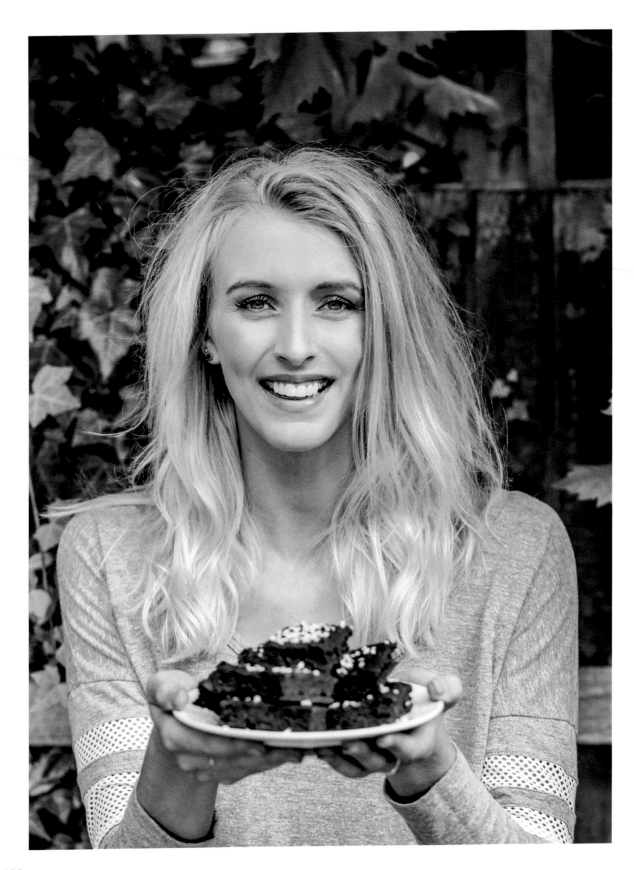

NOURISH

We need to change our perception of food. Many see it as the enemy, something that makes us gain weight and feel guilty. Others see it as a comfort, something to calm us and make everything all right. I see it as fuel. Nourishing, delicious and satisfying fuel. Fuel that our bodies run on. Fuel that can be flavoursome, and fuel to be enjoyed and savoured.

You quite literally are what you eat. Every morsel that passes our lips is broken down by our bodies and used to help us live, breathe, repair, grow and thrive. What we eat affects our organs, muscles, nerves and bones. It can fight disease or fuel disease. It affects how we look, how we feel and how we function. When we open our eyes to this we realise how immensely important food is and we start to see it in a different light. We understand that in order for us to feel energised, become healthier and perform at our best we must fuel ourselves with nourishing, wholesome foods.

However, that doesn't mean that healthy food can't be delicious, or that you can't have chocolate. Let's face it, not many of us can tolerate a diet based purely on kale, green juice and salads, or face the extortionate price tags attached to 'health foods' such as coconut nectar and cacao nibs. The great news is you don't have to! You can achieve amazing results and drastically improve your health while eating delicious, simple food that uses ingredients from your local shop.

I am going to guide you through the basics of nutrition and introduce you to my 'balance principles'. These focus on **wholefoods, colour, flavour, moderation** and **enjoyment**. You won't find any detox recipes, juice cleanses or other radical nonsense. Instead, you will learn how to adopt a simple, balanced approach which gives long-term benefits, and to create quick delicious meals which make you feel amazing.

Gone are the days of restrictive diets, bland meals and low energy levels. It is **your** time to find a sustainable, enjoyable lifestyle full of an abundance of delectable food that makes you feel energised, healthy and glowing. Let me introduce you to just what you need: *balance*!

WHAT YOU REALLY NEED TO KNOW

Before we dive into the principles themselves, here's the low-down on nutrients. I know it can be overwhelming (and boring!), so I am going to avoid the fluff and just give you the key facts.

MACRONUTRIENTS AND MICRONUTRIENTS

Our bodies need nutrients in order to function, and these are categorised as macronutrients or micronutrients. Macronutrients are required in large quantities in order to provide essential nutrients as well as calories which we metabolise for energy: these include proteins, carbohydrates and fats. Micronutrients are just as essential but are required in smaller quantities: these include vitamins and minerals. To put it simply, natural wholefoods such as fruit and vegetables tend to have more micronutrients. Poor-quality processed food, such as cakes and cookies, often contain minimal vitamins and minerals, so are not particularly beneficial to your health. It is essential to eat a balanced and varied diet focusing on wholesome and colourful foods in order to access a wide range of these micronutrients if you want to look, feel and function well.

THE MACRONUTRIENTS

PROTEIN	CARBS	FATS
4 calories per gram	4 calories per gram	9 calories per gram

Alcohol has 7 calories per gram but it isn't an essential macronutrient (nope, not even that Friday afternoon G&T!).

CARBOHYDRATES

Carbohydrates are a class of compounds containing carbon, hydrogen and oxygen. They include monosaccharides (simple sugars, containing a single 'sugar unit'), disaccharides (made up of 2 'sugar units'), oligosaccharides (short chains of 'sugar units') and polysaccharides (long chains of thousands of 'sugar units', including some types of fibre). Carbohydrates can be found in food such as grains, potatoes, fruit, starchy vegetables, legumes and more. They are certainly not the devil and they don't make you fat, despite their bad press. In fact, carbohydrates are the body's main source of energy, and the easiest one for us to break down and use during exercise. They are also required for the functioning of our kidneys, muscles, central nervous system and brain. Don't cut them out of your diet and expect to function well or perform at your best. You wouldn't expect your car to run on empty, so why expect it of your body and mind? As a general rule, the more

The wholewheat myth:

Contrary to popular belief, wholemeal foods are not wholesome foods. They contain a minimal amount of micronutrients and few health benefits compared to more nutrient-dense carbohydrate sources such as potatoes, fruit, starchy vegetables and legumes. Enjoy wholewheat carbohydrates on occasion, but prioritise more natural sources when you can.

Fibre refers to a range of substances, including certain types of carbohydrates, that are not digested in our stomach or small intestine. They pass through to the large intestine, where some types of fibre are fermented or digested by the bacteria there. Other types pass through the digestive system and out of the body. As a group, the different types of fibre provide a host of benefits. These include promoting satiety, improving glycemic control (blood-sugar levels), decreasing blood cholesterol and, of course... helping you poo! I recommend aiming for 30g of fibre a day as a minimum, which can be achieved quite easily through regular consumption of fibrous foods such as vegetables, fruit, legumes and wholegrains.

active you are, the more carbohydrates your body needs. A sedentary individual requires less energy than someone who exercises regularly or who is on their feet all day.

PROTEIN

Protein is a macronutrient that plays an essential role in our bodies. All of the enzymes in our bodies are proteins and, as a result, the many thousands of chemical reactions that rely on enzymes require this macronutrient. A large proportion of our muscles and other body tissues are made up of proteins. Not only is it involved in the structure of cells themselves and the processes of growth and repair, but it contributes to metabolic, immune, transport and hormone systems and is required for the function of digestive organs, glands, tendons and arteries. Basically, it is pretty important.

Proteins are complex compounds made up of many amino acids linked by peptide bonds. Our bodies make amino acids in two different ways: from scratch or by modifying those we get from our diet.

There are 20 amino acids that our body requires. Of these 20, there are 9 that cannot be manufactured by our cells, so they must be consumed through food. Animal protein sources such as meat deliver all these essential amino acids in one package, whereas plant protein sources tend to lack one or more. Vegetarians need to be aware of this and ensure that they eat a variety of protein-rich foods every day in order to access all the amino acids needed to make protein.

In my opinion, protein is the micronutrient which needs to be given the highest priority. As a basic guideline, I recommend including

"Love yourself enough to nourish your body."

a protein source in the majority of your meals and snacks. A good place to start is with an intake of 1.2-1.6g of protein per kilo of bodyweight. As a rule of thumb, the more activity you do and the more muscle mass you gain, the higher your protein intake should be. It can be increased quite easily by upping your protein portion sizes in your meals and snacks. If you're wondering where to get this vital macronutrient, protein can be found in foods such as meat, fish, dairy, legumes, nuts, seeds, quinoa and eggs. So stock your shelves with good-quality sources to ensure you access all of its health benefits!

A diet rich in protein is **not** going to make you turn into The Hulk! It will just help you to recover quickly and efficiently from your workouts. However, although protein is super-important in your diet you should not eat it in excess at the expense of the other macronutrients — carbohydrates and fats. You need to find a balance of all three in order to achieve optimal health benefits.

FAT

Fats are awesome. Not only do they increase satiation and create delectable flavours and textures, they also have health benefits (contrary to their bad reputation). Fats are essential to growth and development, formation of hormones, maintenance of cell membranes and the absorption of fat-soluble vitamins such as A, D, E and K; plus they are an energy source.

Dietary fats are mainly eaten in a form called triglycerides, with over 90% of our dietary fat coming in this form. The rest is comprised of other fatty substances such as cholesterol. The triglycerides are made up of different combinations and structures of fatty acids, which determine whether they are trans fats, monounsaturated fats, polyunsaturated fats or saturated fats. These fats are summarised below:

TRANS FATS These are vegetable oils that go through a process of partial hydrogenation which changes their chemical structure. It is widely accepted that these fats have little to no health benefits, and can in fact be detrimental to your health. They are found in heavily processed food such as shop-bought cakes, biscuits, pies and some margarines.

SATURATED FATS These are solid at room temperature and primarily found in animal sources such as beef, butter and cheese, but also in some plant sources such as coconut oil. They have a bad reputation, as previous health advice suggested they were harmful and linked to heart disease. However, recent research has shown that they may not be as bad as they were believed to be. Firm conclusions in this area are yet to be reached, but for the time being these fats are recommended by the British Heart Foundation to be consumed in moderation.

UNSATURATED FATS These are categorised as monounsaturated and polyunsaturated fats, and are liquid at room temperature. It is generally accepted that these 'healthy fats', such as olive oil, do not have a negative impact on health, and that can in fact give health benefits when consumed from wholefood sources.

Examples include avocados, fish, and nuts. One particularly important type of unsaturated fat that we *need* to consume (as our body can't create it) is Omega-3 fatty acids. These fats are an integral part of cell membranes. They affect the function of cell receptors and play a role in regulating blood clotting. Food containing high levels of these include oil-rich fish, such as salmon, mackerel and sardines. Plant sources, including walnuts and flaxseeds, also contribute some Omega-3 fat.

Fats should not be feared and, despite what the media may tell you, when consumed as part of a healthy and balanced diet they don't make you fat. I recommend prioritising unsaturated fats, consuming saturated fats in moderation and avoiding trans fats when you can. Ensure the majority of your dietary fats come from wholefood sources and try to consume sources of Omega-3 fatty acids on a regular basis. Be careful when consuming 'low fat' foods such as low-fat yoghurt. Often, in order to replicate that full-fat flavour and texture, they can be pumped full of chemicals and sugar.

Egg yolks have a bad reputation due to the higher levels of cholesterol they contain. However, they are not a threat to your heart health unless you have a pre-existing condition. Eating foods rich in cholesterol does not necessarily cause you to have increased levels. In fact, the yolk is where the majority of the egg's goodness is, so don't discard it.

THE MICRONUTRIENTS

VITAMINS

Vitamins are a diverse group of organic compounds. Many vitamins need to be consumed, as our bodies cannot synthesise them. Vitamins are split into two main types:

Fat-soluble vitamins, which require fat for their absorption into the body, including vitamins A, D, E and K. These have functions such as supporting the functioning of the skin, facilitating the absorption of calcium, blood clotting and maintaining muscle structure. These can be stored in the liver and fat tissue so do not need to be consumed every day.

Water-soluble vitamins, which cannot be stored in the body, and as a result need to be consumed more frequently. These include the B vitamins and vitamin C, which play vital roles in energy metabolism and the production of collagen.

MINERALS

Minerals are inorganic, naturally occurring compounds. These are often divided into macrominerals and microminerals. Macrominerals are required in larger quantities by our bodies, and examples include calcium, iron, sodium and magnesium. Microminerals are required in smaller amounts and examples include copper, chromium and selenium. Minerals play a variety of roles in our body such as fluid balance, oxygen transport, nerve transmission and bone health.

REMEMBER...

Vitamins and minerals are absolutely essential for overall health. So how can you make sure you're consuming enough? Just try to eat a varied, balanced and wholesome diet which includes all the macronutrients and food groups, mostly single-ingredient foods and an abundance of fruits and vegetables in a variety of colours. Simple.

WATER

You've heard it before, but water is essential. Our bodies are 50–60% water depending on your gender, which basically makes us human cucumbers! When you drink enough water you function better in a multitude of ways: it improves your mental and physical performance, aids digestion and increases your energy levels. Plus, drinking more water improves satiety and fights cravings (as we often confuse thirst with hunger).

Other than just feeling thirsty, warning signs that you're dehydrated can include dark-yellow strong-smelling urine (sorry for the TMI!), feeling sluggish and light-headed and having a dry mouth.

So, how much water should you be drinking? This is a question that is still under debate. The general guideline is 1.5 litres a day, which is a great place to start and the amount I recommend as a minimum for most people. However, your overall intake will depend on a number of factors, such as your height, age, weight, energy expenditure, diet and the temperature. As a general rule, the more active, sweaty and hot you get, the more you should drink. As you lose fluid, try to replace it by drinking more water and eating fruit and vegetables with a high water content, such as celery, bell peppers and watermelon.

Most of us tend not to drink enough water, so here are my top practical tips to increase your intake:

• Fill a BPA-free 1-litre water bottle, take it everywhere with you and aim to drink the entire contents at least twice a day.

• Place your bottle of water next to your bed at night, and when you wake up aim to drink half of it first thing in the morning.

• Try using a bottle with a straw as it makes sipping water so much more convenient and easy.

• Set reminders on your phone to drink water multiple times a day (there are also apps for this such as My Water Balance).

• If you find water boring, add some chopped fruit, vegetables or fresh herbs to give it flavour. My personal favourite is sliced cucumber and mint leaves.

• Whenever you go out for a coffee or a meal, always order water along with any other beverages.

Top tip: to get the greatest benefits, try to stick to water as much as you can, rather than sweetened tea, coffee or juices. This ensures that you aren't drinking caffeine and calories along with the fluid.

PUTTING IT TOGETHER

So now you know all about the basic macro- and micronutrients, what they are and why we need each of them. Hopefully you now understand how each of them is beneficial to our health and how we function. So many people look to achieve weight loss by cutting out whole macronutrient groups such as carbohydrates or fat without realising all the consequences. In reality, no single macronutrient is to blame for obesity. Eating too much of **any** macronutrient will lead to weight gain due to excessive calories. It is about *achieving your personal balance* of them all.

Did you know? Our body only needs a handful of amino acids and essential fatty acids as well as a selection of vitamins and minerals and sufficient fluid to run its basic processes; it can produce almost everything else itself. However, in order to function effectively, it also requires sufficient calories to provide the energy it needs. These calories can be consumed from a combination of carbohydrates, protein and fats depending on your preferences, and our bodies are flexible in the energy sources they use depending on what is consumed and available.

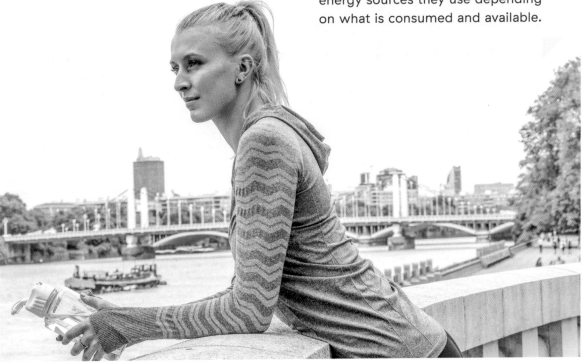

A BRIEF NOTE ON 'TRACKING MACROS'

You may have heard of the term 'tracking macros', which is an approach whereby you calculate exactly how many grams of protein, fats and carbohydrates you want to consume each day to reach your goals. You then weigh and measure all of your food and track it using an app such as MyFitnessPal. I personally don't recommend this approach to many people in the long term. While it is appropriate - and it can be very effective - for bodybuilders, athletes and those who have very specific goals, I think that for the average person it can be a bit of a hassle. It can take up a lot of time (something which we don't have much of!) and make eating socially a challenge. Quite frankly, I don't need another thing on my to-do list and I am sure you don't either. Can you imagine weighing and measuring all your food for the rest of your

life? In front of your kids? In front of your grandkids? In your Zimmer frame? I certainly can't, which is why I think it is essential to become in tune with your body early on, and learn how to eat a balanced diet intuitively.

However, I do think that it can be appropriate to track your dietary intake at the very beginning of your fitness journey. If you are struggling to get to grips with exactly how much food you should be eating, or wondering whether you're getting enough of each macronutrient, tracking your intake just for a week or two can be extremely useful. It can be an eye-opener and give an insight into what you're really consuming and what an appropriate portion size is for you. Also, if later on in your journey you feel like you're getting a bit lost with your eating patterns, you can try tracking for a day or two to check in with yourself.

Let's talk about sugar

Sugar is often seen as the spawn of Satan, the root of all evil and something to be avoided like the plague. In reality, it isn't all that bad. I am only going to touch on it briefly here, as there are whole books devoted to the subject, but my basic principles are these:

• Not all sugar is the same: for example, white processed sugar is empty calories with little nutritional value, whereas the sugar from fruit or some vegetables, such as sweetcorn, contains a whole host of nutrients. If you're going for something sweet, try to choose fruit over cake.

• Stick to whole fruits rather than juices. They have a higher fibre content which can help to slow the

release of the sugar. If you're a fruit fiend then it might be wise to switch a couple of your servings for less sugar–dense fruit such as berries.

• It is all about balance. Too much of anything is an issue. Consuming natural foods that have a higher sugar content is acceptable in moderation, as long as you're not eating dates for breakfast, lunch, dinner and snacks!

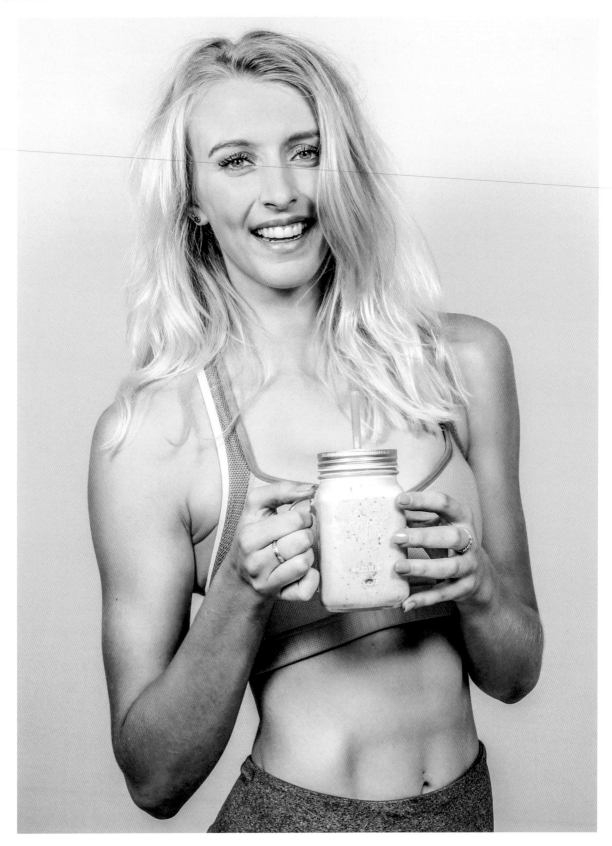

THE BALANCE PRINCIPLES

Let's get down to the nitty gritty. The balance principles are nutrition guidelines that I follow on a daily basis. Read them, absorb them and apply them to your life. I promise that you will feel amazing for it.

FOOD IS FUEL

As a society we have lost connection with what food really is. It is not chemical laden, preservative-covered artificial concoctions moulded to resemble something edible. Food is natural. It is fresh. It is wholesome. It has minimal ingredients. We need to remind ourselves that we absolutely are what we eat. Your body breaks down and uses food to run basic processes, to repair cells and to function effectively. Take a moment to think about that. If you eat refined, processed and poor-quality food all day every day, that is what your body is absorbing and using to make you live. How can you expect to feel good and perform well when your body is running on rubbish? Honestly, you can't.

When you eat a huge pizza and follow it up with an ice cream sundae, how do you really feel? I personally tend to slip into a lethargic food coma and resemble a sloth. I lack energy and have poor concentration levels. These feelings are a sign from our bodies that they are struggling to handle the food we have eaten. We call this comfort food, but is it really comforting?

Food should make you feel awesome. A diet that focuses on colourful wholefoods such as fruit, vegetables, lean proteins, complex carbohydrates and healthy fats will enable your body to run efficiently. When you fuel yourself with wholesome nutrient-dense foods, your body will thank you. It will have an abundance of nutrients available and, as a result, you will thrive from the inside out.

FUEL YOUR WORKOUTS

As you now know, what you eat directly affects how you perform. This brings me swiftly onto pre- and post-workout food: in other words, what you eat before and after a workout. In previous research, a lot of emphasis has been put on these meals and exactly what should be consumed to facilitate optimal recovery and performance. Based on this, I have some general guidelines.

If you train early in the morning and are worrying whether to eat before your workout, there is no single right way. It is essential to find what works for **you**. Try a few different approaches and see how you feel. For some, eating a small carbohydrate-rich snack before their workout makes them feel energised. Others may find this makes them feel sluggish, and that they perform better when they train fasted (that is, without eating beforehand). I prefer to train fasted first thing in the morning, and I find that eating a carbohydrate-rich meal the night before fuels my early workout, and also helps me sleep like a log! If you train later in the day, try to ensure you eat a balanced meal a couple of hours prior to your workout so your stomach has time to settle before you train.

Alright, let's talk about post-workout food. You might have heard of the 'anabolic window', a theory that suggests you need to consume a certain amount of protein within around 30 minutes of a workout or all your gains will be lost. I hate to break it to you, but after 30 minutes your body doesn't instantly turn into a gain-losing machine. There isn't a huge rush to down a protein shake or eat some chicken. In fact, what most affects your results is your diet as a whole, and your overall protein consumption throughout the day. You need to ensure that you're eating enough to support your goals. However, I would recommend that you don't wait all day before eating your post-workout meal (especially if you train fasted first thing in the morning). I would also ensure that the meal includes a combination of protein and carbohydrates, to aid muscle growth and recovery and replenish your muscle glycogen (energy) stores.

TASTE IS KING

Just because food is fuel, doesn't mean it can't also be tasty. Food is not there just to nourish our bodies and make us feel amazing - it can also be damn delicious and provide us with immense pleasure. Gone are the days of grilled chicken, boiled rice and steamed broccoli. Now we can make healthy food indulgent and flavoursome. After all, how can you expect to stick to a balanced diet if you don't enjoy the good food that you're eating? Taste needs to be prioritised! Burritos, brownies and even burgers... you can put healthy twists on all of them, without compromising on flavour. Flick to my recipes on pages 170-243 to find out how.

EAT A RAINBOW

And I don't mean a pack of Skittles!

Plant-based foods like fruit, vegetables, nuts, beans and wholegrains contain phytonutrients (or plant nutrients) such as carotenoids and flavonoids. These are not essential to keep us alive, unlike some vitamins and minerals, but they are linked to a host of health benefits such as improved immune function and a reduced risk of cancer. Many phytonutrients are found in the highest amounts in different coloured fruit and vegetables, so an easy way to access a whole range of them is to eat a 'rainbow' of foods.

Although research in the area of phytonutrients is still developing, it is undeniable that consuming a range of good-quality wholesome food such as fruits and vegetables is going to benefit your overall health. However, a recent UK National Diet and Nutrition survey showed that only 30% of adults aged 19-64 reach the recommended five portions of fruit and vegetables a day - a shocking statistic. My own feeling is that the recommendation of five a day isn't enough. Scrap that and go for more. I say 6 or 7 portions or more is ideal, with 4 to 5 of these being vegetables. Fruit and vegetables are, for the most part, low in calories and high in nutrients, so eat them in abundance.

I know that my recommendations can sound daunting, especially if you're currently averaging a couple of portions of fruit and veg a day. So here are some practical tips to increase your intake:

• It seems obvious, but buy more fruit and veg. Try to step out of your comfort zone and choose unfamiliar ones that you haven't cooked with before. You never know, you might find a new favourite.

• Get a fruit bowl, fill it with whichever fruits you like best and pop it on your table or kitchen worktop – anywhere where it is readily available or in sight. This means that next time you're looking for a snack, you will see the fruit first, before the chocolate bars in your cupboard.

• Add fruit and vegetables to your smoothies and shakes. I love adding frozen banana to protein shakes to give them the texture of ice cream, and a handful of spinach for a serving of greens (which I promise you can't taste).

• Bulk up your meals. I always add a host of vegetables to curries, chilli, Bolognese, soups and more. If you chop them finely they don't interfere with the flavour or texture, they simply add a boost of nutrients.

• When you're in a hurry just throw together a stir fry (see page 191). Stir fries are a one-pan wonder which take 5 minutes to cook. Shove a bunch of veg and some meat into a pan with spices, cook them through and bish bash bosh, you have a nourishing meal.

• Pimp your salads. I'm lazy... I'm certainly guilty of shoving some meat and spinach in a bowl and calling it a salad. Salads are so much more than lettuce leaves and can be varied and delicious. Try squeezing in *at least* 3 different vegetables and don't be afraid to add fruit: why not try my Smoked Salmon, Mango and Pistachio Salad on page 193? Yum!

• Prepare for snack attacks. Keep fruit and vegetables in your handbag or on your desk ready for those mid-afternoon cravings.

• Mix up your omelettes. Omelettes are a perfect base for cramming in some veg. Just add all your favourite greens along with some spices (and maybe a cheeky bit of cheese) and prepare for a seriously yummy meal.

• Eat dessert. And that's an order! Fruit is an amazing dessert and you can really get creative with it. For example, blitz two frozen bananas with a dash of milk in a blender to create home-made ice cream or bake apples and plums and stuff them with berries for a warming treat.

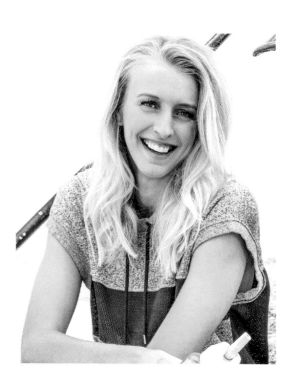

WHAT COUNTS AS A PORTION?

FRUIT	VEGETABLES
1 large slice of melon	7 asparagus spears
1 banana	1 dessert bowl of salad
1 apple	½ a pepper/courgette/aubergine
2 satsumas/kiwis/plums	2 large broccoli spears
1 heaped tablespoon of raisins	1 onion/leek/parsnip
2 handfuls of berries	3 heaped tablespoons of pulses e.g. beans & peas

CONSIDER INGREDIENTS

Natural food doesn't have a label. Think of nutritious foods such as fruit, vegetables, salmon, potatoes, rice, olive oil – they don't have a list of ingredients. You don't need to look at what is in a banana, a carrot or an egg. You don't need to worry about them having added nasties. These are **single-ingredient foods**. Now think about shop-bought cakes, biscuits and ice cream. They usually all have long ingredient lists, which often include things we can't pronounce or don't recognise. They are often laden with added colours, preservatives and thickeners to enhance their flavour and texture and extend their shelf life. Do you really want to put these into your body?

I'm not saying that you can't consume any food that contains additives. That stuff is designed to be delicious. Just eat these things in moderation and ensure that you prioritise natural, single-ingredient wholefoods in the majority of your meals. Also, in recent times there has been a shift towards the development of more natural pre-prepared foods. When browsing the aisles of your local supermarket you can come across energy balls, fresh sauces and various other products, all of which have minimal ingredients. Just make sure you don't accept at face value the 'all natural' or 'healthy' marketing splashed across a multitude of packaging. Check the label yourself.

Top tip: As someone whose parents are growers, I understand how vital it is to support local farmers and businesses. When you can, try to source your meat, dairy and produce from local markets, butchers and delis. Not only does this support your community but it means you get access to the freshest ingredients. It's a win–win situation.

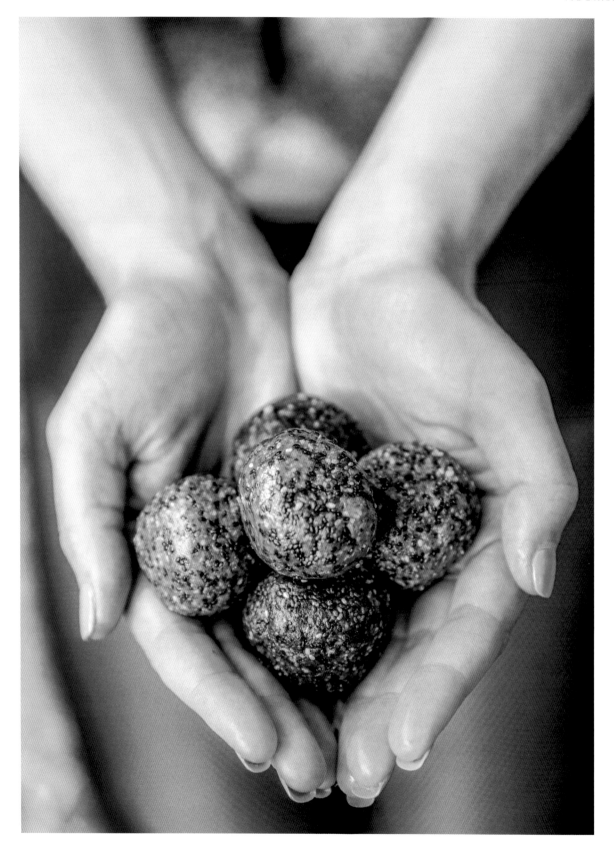

COOK FROM SCRATCH

I understand that every so often you can find yourself in a sticky situation and needing to grab a pre-made salad or sarnie. But on the whole, I recommend trying to make the vast majority of your meals yourself. Prepared food often has added ingredients that aren't always the best for you and your goals. When you cook for yourself, you know exactly what is going into your body and you take responsibility for the results. Now, you might well be thinking: 'But I hate cooking' or 'I don't have time'. My mission with this book is to show you that healthy food can be quick to make, simple and delicious. Making balanced, nourishing and tasty meals is achievable. Here are my top tips to fit it into your life:

• Make it social. Kill two birds with one stone by combining socialising with cooking. Grab a friend, choose a recipe and cook together. It is also an amazing and productive way to spend time with your other half.

• Use your weekends wisely. Weekends are a great time to sneak in some meal prep. Try cooking up a big batch of Bolognese, grilling some chicken breasts or throwing together a couple of huge salads. Store them in the fridge in airtight containers and eat them during the first half of the week, or freeze single servings of the Bolognese or chicken breasts for later.

• Prepare breakfast the night before. If you're always in a hurry in the morning, try making your breakfast in advance. It takes 5 minutes to put together a bowl of Overnight Oats (see page 172) or pop your smoothie ingredients in a blender (see page 174). Then you can grab and go!

• Cook in batches. When you prepare an evening meal, try to make more than you're going to eat. Keep the leftovers and pop them in a lunchbox for the next day or two.

• Identify your staple meals. These are meals that take you minimal time to make but are balanced and delicious. They are your backup plan for when you're seriously short on time. My personal favourites are simple stir-fries (see my Basic Chicken Stir Fry on page 191), zoats (see my Cinnamon Spice Protein Zoats on page 173) and omelettes.

• Let the cooker do the work. I mean the slow-cooker. These things are seriously useful. Just throw in some meat, vegetables and stock (preferably the low-salt variety) in the morning and come home to a meal that is ready to be eaten. Simple.

YOU DON'T NEED TO CUT OUT EVERYTHING

Everywhere I look, I see food labelled 'gluten-free', 'dairy-free', 'fat-free' or 'sugar-free'. There is a serious trend for cutting out food groups, a trend I think needs to stop. No single food, nutrient or ingredient is the root of all evil.

Gluten and dairy get blamed for everything and anything, but are they really that bad? If you are legitimately allergic or intolerant to them, they can be. However, the vast majority of us have no issues with consuming and digesting them, so have no need to avoid them. My only advice is to stick to the most wholesome sources you can, such as less processed dairy products and home-made or locally made wholegrain or granary bread.

You need to listen to your body. The better your digestion, the better your absorption of nutrients. If you are having any digestive issues or discomfort after eating, please go to your doctor. Do not self-diagnose. A qualified professional can identify any medical issues and help you to resolve them.

Another important thing to note is that when something is labelled 'free from' a certain ingredient, it does not mean it is healthy. For example, fat-free yoghurt is often pumped full of added sugar, while gluten-free cake can be as calorie-dense and nutrient-poor as regular cake. When you remove an ingredient you often have to add something else to give the food product the same flavour and texture as the original version. Get your cynical pants on, read the label and make an informed decision.

CALORIES MATTER

Ultimately, calories **do** matter and we have to balance our energy expenditure. If we eat more food than we require and don't move our bodies on a regular basis, then we will be in a caloric surplus and our body fat will increase. If we move more and eat in a slight caloric deficit, we will become leaner. And if we eat the amount of food our bodies require for maintenance, and train consistently, then we can become fitter, stronger and healthier! However, calorie counting and macro tracking are time-consuming approaches and can be unsustainable in the long term. Instead, I like to control my intake by focusing on portions and ensuring that my meals and servings are an appropriate size for fuelling my body.

WHAT SHOULD BE ON YOUR PLATE?

As a general recommendation, when preparing your own meals try to include a portion all three macronutrients; carbohydrates, proteins and fats. The table overleaf outlines some example portion sizes but it is also useful to look at hand measurements or consider the size of the plate itself when working out your servings.

Please note: these hand measurements are rough guidelines and don't apply to all foods in each category, as can be seen in the table on page 144.

- **Protein:** Roughly a palm-sized amount or a quarter of your plate.

- **Carbohydrates:** Roughly a palm-sized amount or a quarter of your plate.

- **Fats:** Roughly a thumb-sized portion.

- **Greens & Veggies:** These are unlimited; I recommend aiming for half of your plate to be filled with them. What counts as greens? It's not just salad – greens also include fibrous vegetables such as broccoli, green beans, courgettes, spinach, kale, pak choi, asparagus and cucumber. Examples of other veggies you could try include bell peppers, onions, red cabbage and carrots.

ADAPTING THESE PORTIONS

These guidelines are based on an average Joe and are a great place to start. However it is vital to adapt portion sizes to your body, goals, activity levels and preferences. Here are some basic adaptions:

Your preferences: I recommend consuming a protein source at most (if not all) main meals. However, the amount of carbohydrates and fats you consume is in your hands. I have

EXAMPLE 'SINGLE PORTION' SERVING SIZES

These examples illustrate the variety of different foods you can consume to access each macronutrient, and simple portion sizes.

PROTEIN	CARBOHYDRATES	FATS
2 eggs	½ cup cooked rice or quinoa	½ an avocado
1 chicken breast	1 medium sweet potato	1 tbsp peanut butter (or the whole jar if you're like me...)
1 salmon fillet	½ cup dry oats	1 tbsp olive oil
125g beef mince	1 slice wholegrain bread	1 small handful of nuts
150g chickpeas, lentils or beans	1 banana	A thumb-sized piece of cheese
1 scoop of good quality whey or vegan protein powder	Unlimited vegetables	⅓ cup full-fat natural yoghurt

It should be noted that the vast majority of these foods cross the boundaries between the macronutrient groups such as legumes containing protein and carbohydrates, and yoghurt containing a substantial amount of protein as well fat. Be sure to read the label.

outlined basic serving recommendations but these can vary between meals. So if you fancy a more carb-heavy meal for breakfast and a fatty meal for lunch, then go for it! Just try to keep a good balance across the whole day.

Your body: The bigger your body, the more food it requires. Tall people like me tend to need more fuel to keep them going, whereas more petite people need less. The more muscle mass you have, the higher your resting metabolism, which means you can consume more calories (my favourite reason to lift weights!).

Your activity level: The more active you are, the more calories you burn and the more food

you can eat (now that's a great excuse to work out!). If you have a very active job and are on your feet all day, you will need more fuel than if you sit at a desk for 8 hours. If you have a particularly physical day then be sure to eat enough food to fuel your body.

Your goals: Your portions will depend on whether you want to lose weight, maintain your weight or gain weight, with smaller portions for weight loss and larger portions for weight gain.

So, if you're a petite, inactive individual you will be eating fewer calories than a highly active, tall individual. It is far too easy to

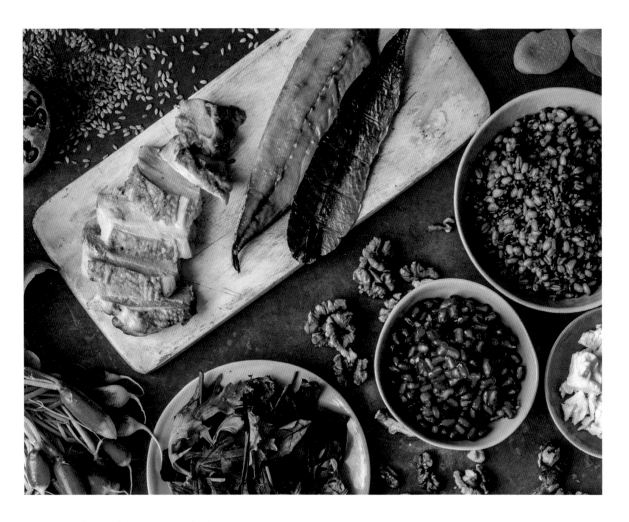

overestimate how many calories we are burning, and underestimate how many calories we are eating. As a result, we can easily overeat energy-rich foods when in reality we aren't using that much energy.

It is essential to be honest and realistic with yourself about how much activity you do. This is where fitness trackers can come in useful. I recommend starting with my basic guidelines, making adaptions based on your personal situation and preferences, see how your body reacts and how you feel, and go from there. Don't stress about it, go with the flow and find what works for **you**.

Calories and portion sizes are clearly key factors in determining your energy levels, performance and your results. However, many other elements are also influencing your body and mind, such as your hormone functioning. If you have a medical condition or are experiencing any unusual symptoms, then be sure to visit your doctor who can clarify how this might affect your health and fitness journey.

SNACKS

It is very easy to overeat when it comes to snacks, so I really try to control my portion sizes and ensure they don't become mini meals. Here are a few examples of well-portioned healthy snacks:

• A portion of fruit e.g. a banana, a handful of berries, half a mango. (My favourites are a chopped apple topped with ground cinnamon or fresh mango with lime juice squeezed on top!)

• 2 rice cakes topped with 1 tablespoon of nut butter and few berries.

• A protein shake with 1 scoop of protein powder, half a banana and milk of your choice.

• A few of pieces of chocolate.

• 2 tablespoons of natural nut butter (out of the jar!).

• ⅓ cup natural yoghurt topped with berries.

• A handful of nuts.

• 1 home-made protein bar, brownie or granola bar.

• 3 small home-made energy balls.

• 2 cups of popcorn sprinkled with cinnamon.

• Veggies dipped in a couple of tablespoons of humous.

• 1 small home-made chia pudding.

Dealing with snack attacks

I am a serial snacker. I want to eat all day every day and can find myself grazing on anything and everything. The thing is, snacks add up quickly and can lead to overeating, so you need to be careful. Here are my top tips for when the cravings kick in:

• First things first, drink a big glass of water. We often mistake thirst for hunger, meaning dehydration can make us feel peckish. If you're still hungry 20 minutes later, have a snack.

• Ask yourself a question: can I eat an apple instead? If the answer is no, you're not really that hungry and are just eating for the sake of it. If the answer is yes, then go ahead and eat one, or have another equally as nutritious snack.

• Make healthy snacking convenient. Keep a fruit bowl in clear view and vegetable sticks chopped up in the fridge. Pop your cakes, biscuits and crisps in harder-to-reach places.

• Eat smart. Just because something is 'healthy' doesn't mean you can eat your bodyweight in it. For example, raw brownies are made from all-natural ingredients, but they can be up to 300 calories a slice, so watch your portions.

SLOW AND STEADY WINS THE RACE

You might have read the previous section and thought, 'Damn, I need to drastically reduce my portion sizes'. Don't panic, you don't. If you cut your calories significantly right from the beginning you're setting yourself up for deprivation and failure.

Like I said, food is fuel. If you go straight in and substantially reduce your portions and calories, you will feel the consequences. Your energy levels will drop and, as a result, so will your functioning and performance. Plus, you're more likely to plateau (stop losing weight) as your body will adapt to the changes you made meaning you will need to eat less and less food to continue making progress, which isn't ideal. The smaller the caloric changes, the better.

It is essential to take it slowly to achieve lasting results. I recommend focusing on making healthy swaps and increasing your intake of wholesome rather than processed foods **before** you start specifically controlling portions. By nature, wholesome single-ingredient foods are higher in nutrients and lower in calories than refined processed foods, which are lower in nutrients and higher in calories. So, if you swap your French fries for baked sweet potato wedges or your chocolate bar for a piece of fruit, then you're already reducing your overall caloric intake. By focusing your meals around a variety of vegetables, lean proteins, wholegrain carbohydrates and portion-controlled healthy fats you will naturally reduce calories and increase nutrients.

Remember, being in a caloric deficit isn't something you can do forever, so if you're aiming to get leaner you need to stay savvy. Once you have reached your goal, be sure to slowly bring your portions back up to maintenance levels; this means an amount of food which you can comfortably eat to maintain your weight and support optimal functioning.

MY LITTLE SECRET... VOLUME EATING

I eat with my eyes. I like having a full plate or bowl of food. It is a psychological thing: serving up a plate that is full to the brim with delicious ingredients makes us feel more satisfied. However, this is my downfall, as it can easily lead to me overeating without even realising it, *oops*!

An easy way to eat more food for fewer calories is by looking at caloric density. Consider one Oreo. It weighs 11 grams and totals 52 calories. Compare this to spinach, where to get 52 calories you would need around 200 grams, which is practically a mountain of it! Which one will make you feel good? Which one will fuel your body more effectively? The spinach. I admit I don't want to eat a bag of the stuff in one go, but you get my point! As I said, wholesome foods are high in nutrients and low in calories, plus they're full of fibre which keeps you feeling fuller for longer. Eat them in abundance.

I will let you in on my secret. The reason I can still eat mountains of food is because I 'volume eat'. This means I bulk up meals with these nutrient-dense, low-calorie foods, chiefly vegetables. There are obvious ways you can do this: making huge salads for example, or roasting a heap of colourful vegetables and adding these to your meals. There are also less obvious ways, and that's where it gets interesting. Here are my favourite sneaky volume eats:

COURGETTE

Ahhh, the humble courgette. The miracle vegetable which is so often underestimated. The most popular way to use courgette these days is as 'courgetti' – in other words, courgette spaghetti. This is where you slice the vegetable into spaghetti-like strips using a spiralizer or a julienne peeler and use it to bulk out or replace pasta. However, did you know you can grate it and add it to your porridge? It massively increases your serving size, gives you a nutritious serving of greens and adds minimal calories. Want to know how? Check out my Cinnamon Spice Protein Zoats recipe on page 173.

CAULIFLOWER AND BROCCOLI

These two nutrient-dense powerhouses can be made into rice. Use a food processor to whizz them into rice-size pieces (or grate them if you have the time and patience), then stir-fry with spices of your choice. You can add this to rice to bulk it out, or serve it alone as an alternative.

SPAGHETTI SQUASH

As the name suggests, this squash provides an amazing plant-based spaghetti. Slice the squash in half lengthways, remove the seeds and rub oil of your choice on the non-skin surfaces (I recommend coconut oil). Place it cut side down on a baking sheet and bake at 180°C/350°F/Gas Mk 4 for 45 minutes to 1 hour. It is ready when a fork easily pokes through the outer skin. Then use a fork to scoop out the 'spaghetti'. Again, you can use this to bulk out pasta or as an alternative.

POPCORN

You know those days when you just can't stop eating? Try snacking on popcorn. A huge serving (2 cups!) of home-popped popcorn totals well under 100 calories and seriously satisfies cravings. Just buy some of the kernels and pop them at home. Add flavour with salt or cinnamon and stevia (a plant-based sweetener).

ICE

Unsatisfied by your smoothie or shake? Just add ice. Whenever I make any cold blended drink I always add much more ice and less liquid than you would expect. What results is a gigantic thick (and super creamy if you add half a frozen banana) smoothie that is immensely filling and delicious.

Top tip: Another way to trick your mind into thinking you're eating more is to invest in smaller bowls and plates. This means we can serve up less but still feel like we are eating more by filling the dish. This helps you to control your intake without you even realising it!

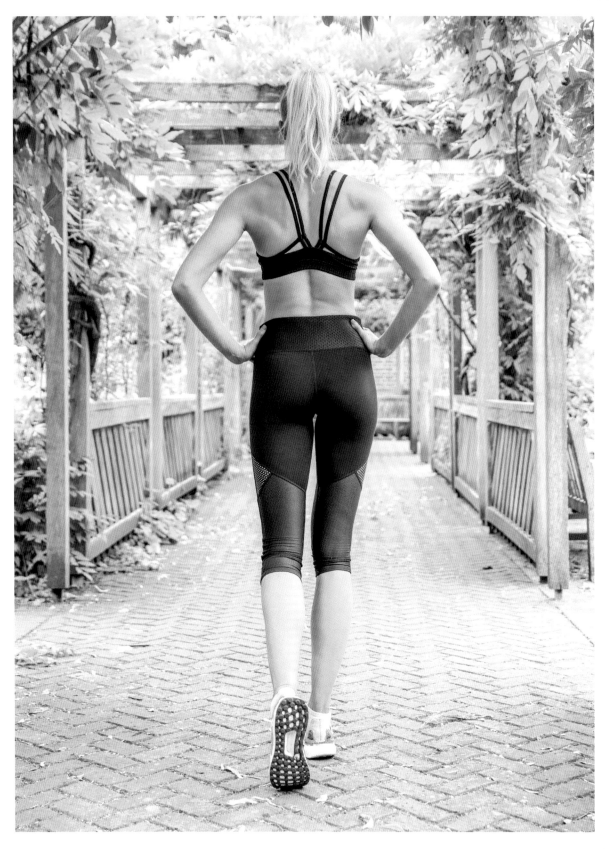

MODERATION IS KEY

What if I told you that you can eat chocolate and pizza and still be healthy? It's true. A balanced approach to living a healthy lifestyle does not cut out anything, especially not the foods you love. It's all about **moderation not deprivation**.

So what does that mean? I like to use the 80/20 rule. This dictates that 80% of your diet is made up of balanced, nutrient-dense meals providing a spectrum of macro and micronutrients. The remaining 20% of your diet is more flexible. You can use this to allow yourself some of your favourite less-wholesome foods. By allowing yourself an occasional treat, you're keeping yourself sane and avoiding any feelings of deprivation, reducing the chance of bingeing or overeating.

What does that 20% equate to? Well that depends on your preferences and lifestyle. For some it might be a small biscuit or mini chocolate bar every day; for others it may be a cheeky burger and a beer on the weekend. It is important to find your own personal balance and what **your** 20% is made up of.

BUT WHAT IF I WANT TO GO COLD TURKEY?

Fair enough, good on you for being so motivated! If you want to cut out all refined and processed foods, then go for it. I certainly think that it can work in the short term, especially if you're new to this lifestyle and really want to kickstart the journey. However, my concern with this approach is that you may end up feeling deprived and having issues with eating out socially. As a result, I recommend a 90/10 approach for the first month or two if you really want to go in at the deep end. Then, once you have established

these healthy habits in your life, you can adapt your diet to follow the 80/20 rule – a more sustainable approach in the long term.

YOU DON'T NEED A MOUNTAIN OF SUPPLEMENTS

When you walk into any health-food shop you will see stacks of every supplement under the sun, from horny goat weed through to raspberry ketones. It can be overwhelming and confusing, not to mention expensive. They promise everything from increased energy levels through to miraculous fat burning. I hate to burst their marketing bubble but we don't need 99% of these tablets as long as we maintain a healthy and balanced diet.

So what **do** we need? Not that much. If you're eating a wholesome diet, you should be able to access most vitamins and minerals. However, there are a handful of supplements I take and recommend you check out:

FISH OILS

Fish oils don't sound glamorous or delicious, and indeed they aren't. However, they are an amazing source of Omega-3 fatty acids, which are linked to increased heart health and reduced inflammation, and which we often lack in our diets. Ideally we should consume these through our diet, but if you don't eat oily fish regularly, a supplement is a great alternative. The most important thing to look for when buying these oils is the levels of active ingredients EPA and DHA, which are specific fatty acids. I recommend taking enough capsules a day that you achieve a minimum of 1g of EPA/DHA. It varies between brands.

VITAMIN D

Ahhh, the elusive vitamin D. This vitamin is not very easy to access through food; our body makes it through exposure of the skin to sunlight. Since most of us spend the majority of our time inside and get minimal sun exposure, it is fairly common to have a vitamin D deficiency. If you are at risk of low sun exposure or spend the majority of your time at a desk indoors, then a standard dose of 10 micrograms per day during the autumn and winter months is a great place to start.

PROTEIN POWDERS

These stand somewhere between a supplement and a food. Ideally you would get all of your protein from wholefood sources such as meat, eggs, beans and dairy. However, powders provide a quick, easy and convenient way for busy people to consume more protein. They should not be heavily relied on but they are especially useful when you're travelling or on-the-go; and they can be used in creative ways in oatmeal, cakes and smoothies, for example. Contrary to popular belief, they don't make you bulky. Think about it like this: having a 30g scoop of protein powder is equivalent to eating a chicken breast.

When choosing a protein powder I recommend finding one with minimal ingredients, a low sugar content, around 15-25g of protein and a great taste. Lots of brands do single-serving sachets you can try before committing to a big tub. For dairy eaters, try a whey protein powder for a protein source containing all the essential amino acids you need. For vegans, there are lots of dairy-free options on the market. Instead of going for a pure pea, hemp or rice protein, try searching for a blend that provides all the essential amino acids to help promote optimal protein synthesis. It is important to note that vegan protein powders often contain higher levels of carbohydrates, so be sure to read the label.

Let me take this opportunity to touch on protein bars. Protein bars *are not* a health food. Manufacturers like to market them as such, but don't be misled. If you take the time to look at their ingredients, they are often as poor quality and low in nutrients as regular chocolate and snack bars. Make sure you read the label and consume them in moderation.

REMEMBER…

Consult a doctor before you start taking any supplements. I'd also suggest getting some basic blood work done at the same time to check for any deficiencies. Some particularly common ones are low iron levels in women, low vitamin D levels in winter, low magnesium levels in those who train heavily, low calcium levels if you avoid dairy and low zinc levels if you avoid red meat. These deficiencies can easily be resolved by taking the relevant supplement as recommended by your health professional.

And while we're talking about supplements…

I want to dispel some of the myths surrounding detox teas and juice cleanses. Brands claim that these help your body to 'reset' and your liver to 'detox your system' which somehow turns you into a mystical creature who rapidly loses weight, develops a flat tummy and has glowing skin. But your body is perfectly capable of detoxing itself; that is the liver's job and it is pretty damn good at it. As long as you drink enough water, it will get on with the job perfectly well on its own.

Mindful Eating

I strongly believe that food is to be savoured. We are often in such a rush that we eat on the go and at our desks or laptops. We do it subconsciously and don't even realise what we are putting into our bodies. How often have you opened a bag of crisps or a packet of biscuits while watching TV and before you know it you've finished them? Eating mindlessly means that we don't enjoy our food as much as we could, and we can overeat more easily.

I highly recommend that you try to eat the majority of your meals in a mindful way. What does this mean? It means taking time enjoy your food. Focus on it away from distractions. Put your phone in airplane mode, close your laptop and turn off the TV. Sit at a table and focus on what you're eating. Don't rush, take your time, notice the flavours and textures. Not only does this allow you to enjoy and appreciate your food

more, but it also prompts you to eat more slowly and allows you to become satisfied more quickly. It makes you aware of what you're consuming and reduces the risk of overeating.

Mindful eating is an important step towards learning to listen to your body and eat intuitively — skills I believe are essential to master. We all have routines engrained through years of social conditioning, such as feeling like we always need to finish the food on our plate, eat dessert or have a mid-afternoon snack. Recognise that many of our eating patterns are habits. You don't have to follow these. It takes time, but we need to become in tune with our bodies and listen to them. If you're hungry then you're hungry. If you're full then you're full. Listen to what your body is trying to tell you. Close your eyes and ask what it really wants. I bet you it's not that seventh slice of pizza.

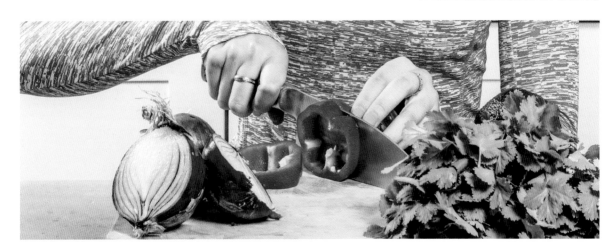

YOU CAN MAINTAIN A SOCIAL LIFE

A common misconception when adopting a healthy lifestyle is that you have to stop eating out and enjoying a glass of wine with friends. That is just untrue. Sure, food is fuel, but food is also a delicious, enjoyable and hugely social thing. Going out to eat is an amazing way to explore a city, try something new or spend time with friends; it shouldn't be feared. That said, I do have a few top tips for staying on track while eating socially:

• Don't arrive hungry. You'll want to eat anything and everything on menu, making it harder to choose wisely. Try having a light snack a couple of hours beforehand to tide you over.

• On a similar note, look at the menu before you arrive if you can and plan what you are going to eat. This means that you can think clearly rather than being swayed by your friends telling you to go for the pizza and chips.

• Pass on the bread basket. If your friends don't mind, you could avoid having a bread basket at all, to help you avoid temptation.

• Focus on getting lean protein in your main course and fill up your plate with salad and fresh veg.

• Try to avoid dishes that are described as 'creamy', 'crispy' or 'fried', as these foods tend not to be prepared in the healthiest of ways. Instead look for grilled or steamed where you can.

• Ask for sauces to be served separately, as these are usually laden with cream and oil.

• Try to go for either a starter or a dessert rather than both.

• Sharing is caring. If you can't resist eating all three courses, try sharing one of them with your dining companion.

• Don't be afraid to ask questions about how the food is prepared or to ask for alterations to the menu. Most restaurants are more than happy to help with any dietary requirements.

• Look at what you're drinking, as drinks are often laden with hidden calories. For example, a coffee with milk, syrup and cream can total over 400 calories. A large glass of wine has around 180 calories and cocktails can range from 100 to over 500 calories apiece. For lighter alternatives stick to water, an espresso or clear spirits with low-calorie tonic.

WHILE WE'RE TALKING ABOUT ALCOHOL...

Alcohol has no nutritional or health benefits, especially when consumed in excess. However, its consumption is a huge part of modern society and I am not going to pretend that everyone is willing to go teetotal. All I am asking is that you be honest with yourself and look at how much you're drinking. I certainly would not recommend drinking more than once or twice a week, and when you do drink, try to stick to one or two lighter options. Try a clear spirit with a diet mixer or my healthy-ish cocktails on pages 242–243. I know it's not what you want to hear, but drinking alcohol regularly can easily ruin your progress, and it certainly isn't nourishing your body.

PUT IT IN CONTEXT...

How healthy and controlled you need to be with your choices depends massively on how often you eat socially. If you're someone who dines out several times a week, you really do need to be careful about what you're consuming. Restaurants do not consider your health and fitness goals when designing their menus, so you need to choose wisely. However, if you eat out once every couple of weeks, then you can be much more flexible. Having a pizza or burger with a glass of wine every once in a while isn't going to throw you off track, so don't be afraid to indulge. Again, be honest with yourself and find your own personal balance.

Top tip: If you are going out for an epic meal or planning on consuming a significant amount of alcohol one evening (I'm not judging you...), try the 'buffer' method. This involves eating a lighter breakfast and lunch to 'save space' for your more indulgent dinner and/or drinks. This **does not** mean severely restricting or starving yourself completely. It simply means making lighter nutrient-dense choices throughout the day to enable you to make less-nutritious choices in the evening.

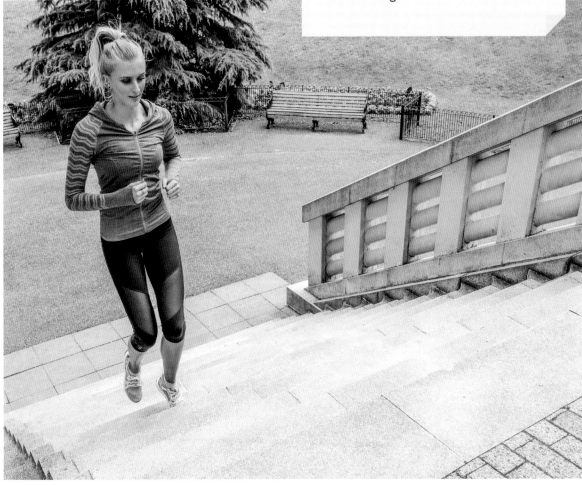

Resisting Temptation

Some people don't like it when their friends, colleagues or family members eat healthily. They try to throw them off track by insisting they have a slice of cake, a bag of crisps or a cheeky cocktail. Sadly, being healthy isn't cool (yet!) and it can be tough to stick to your guns when everyone else is tucking into the office chocolate box. However, I do have some top tips to help you stay strong:

• Keep healthy snacks on hand, whether that's in your handbag or desk drawer. Then, if someone offers you a biscuit when you're hungry, you know that you already have a healthy option available.

• Ask your friends, colleagues or partner to help you stay accountable by reminding you to stay on track, or even try to rope them into joining you on your fitness journey.

• If someone's particularly pushy then have an honest conversation with them. Don't insult their choices or become defensive. Just explain why you're making healthy choices and ask them kindly to respect your decisions.

• When it comes to alcohol, you can be sneaky. Just order a diet soft drink and then when someone asks what you're drinking tell a white lie and say it has a spirit in. No one will ever know as long as they don't take a sip!

• Have an excuse. If a friend is insisting you share a slice of cake with her and you don't want to indulge, it's wise to have an excuse to fall back on, such as 'I've only just eaten'.

• Finally, don't be ashamed of your healthy lifestyle. Keep in mind why you're making these balanced choices. It's for your health and results, not for anyone else. This matters more than other people's opinions, so stay strong and stick to your guns.

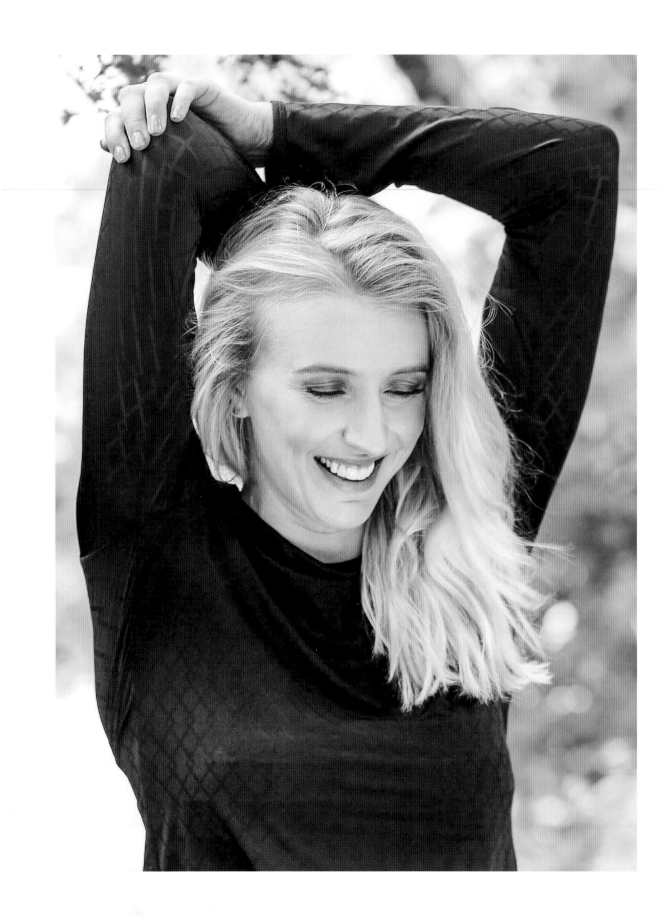

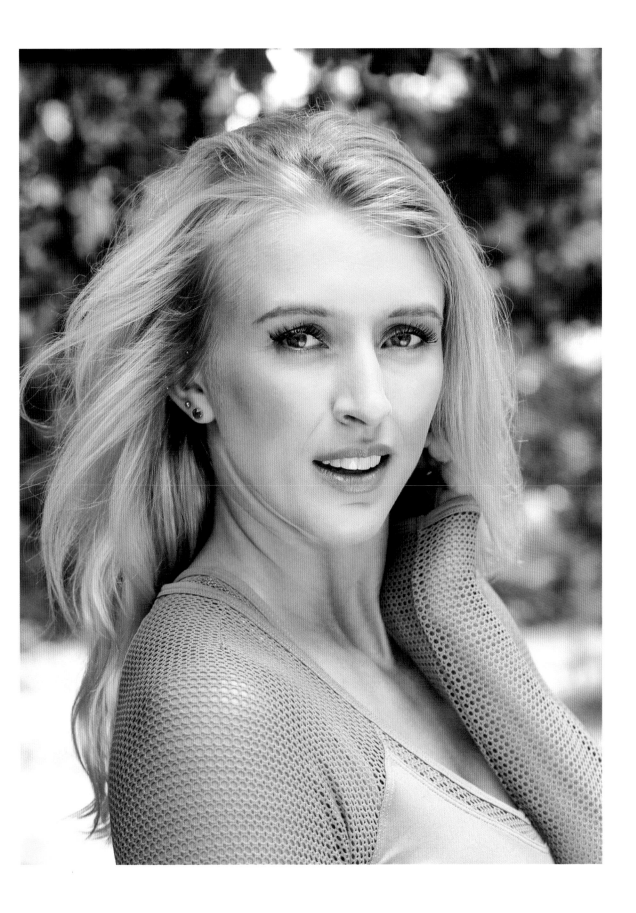

YOU CAN EAT ON THE GO

Now I am **always** going to recommend cooking your own food from scratch when you can. Take it back to your childhood, get some Tupperware and make yourself a yummy packed lunch. It seems like a chore in the beginning, but once you've done it a couple of times it becomes a quick and efficient routine which you know is helping you work towards your goals.

However, I know that sometimes you can be in a sticky situation and have to buy something from the nearest grab-and-go café. I want to ensure that you make the healthiest choices possible in these situations, so here are my top tips:

• High-street food outlets and cafés may seem like the obvious choice, but they can often be more expensive and have fewer healthy options than some supermarkets. You will be surprised by what's available in your local Sainsbury's or Tesco.

• Often on-the-go meals are heavy on one macronutrient (usually refined carbohydrates) and lacking in others, which is why I recommend prioritising protein and greens to avoid any nasties. However, if you can, try to find a balanced option containing lean protein, complex carbohydrates, healthy fats and a variety of veggies.

• My favourite tactic when buying a healthy lunch is to get a pack of pre-cooked meat (usually chicken), a mixed salad bowl and a piece of fruit. I simple pop the chicken in the salad bowl and eat the fruit on the side. Easy.

• Lots of high-street food outlets are now offering 'protein pots' containing eggs or meat with greens. These are a great light snack or component of a healthy lunch.

• Look at the menu online if you can, as some lunch spots don't list the calories or nutritional values in store. This can mean you unwittingly make a less balanced choice. For example, the one particular high-street chain well known for being a healthy lunch station, packs almost 800 calories into its meatball wrap. If you served this with a side of peas at 161 calories and green shake at 136 calories, you would total over 1000 calories in a single meal. Ouch!

• Wherever possible, avoid the meal deals. They may seem cost efficient but they often include crisps, chocolate bars and fizzy drinks. What's more, they can encourage you to buy more food than you need.

• So what should you choose? Try to avoid pies, sandwiches, wraps and sushi. These tend to be heavy on the carbs and light on protein, greens and micronutrients. Try focusing on the salads, soup and hot pots. If you're struggling to make a decision, take a closer look at the labels.

LABELS ARE YOUR BEST FRIENDS

When you're eating on the go, reading labels is absolutely essential. Luckily, it is much easier to understand them nowadays. Most food is clearly labeled with detailed nutritional breakdowns and 'traffic light' illustrations to highlight healthier and less-balanced options. Use this information to inform your decisions.

HOW TO READ A FOOD LABEL

count as one of your 5-a-Day. ...2.3g Fat and 155mg of ...med
adding a handful of fruit will

Typical values	100g contains	45g serving contains
Energy	1570kJ	710kJ
	375kcal	170kcal
Protein	10.3g	4.6g
Carbohydrate	73.8g	33.2g
of which sugars	15.0g	6.8g
Fat	2.0g	0.9g
of which saturates	0.3g	0.1g
Fibre‡‡	8.2g	
Sodium		

INGREDIENTS Less is more when it comes to ingredients. If there is a huge paragraph with lots of long, complex words you can't pronounce, it isn't a good sign. Try to stick to options with short ingredient lists that comprise natural components which you recognise. The largest ingredient is listed first, so if it is sugar, oil or cream, then watch out.

SERVINGS Always check your servings. Often a recommended serving size on a packet is smaller than you might think. Also, brands can be sneaky and put two servings into one small bag, meaning you unwittingly eat more than you intended. To be safe, I like to buy single servings when it is cost-efficient, to avoid overeating.

CALORIES Always check the calories per serving and evaluate how this fits into your full day of eating and level of activity. For example, if you know you're having a large dinner then go lighter with your lunch choice.

PROTEIN In a main meal I recommend trying to hit a minimum of 15g of protein – ideally 20-25g if possible.

CARBOHYDRATES Your carbohydrate intake depends on how you're feeling, how much energy you require, your preferences and how hungry you are. I generally recommend anywhere from 20g of carbohydrates up to 50g or more per serving, depending on your needs.

FATS I recommend aiming for *around* 10-15g of fats per meal, with most of these being unsaturated.

FIBRE Your fibre intake will correlate to your vegetable and carbohydrate intake. I try to hit 7-9g of fibre per meal as a minimum.

SODIUM Try to stick to less than 700 milligrams of sodium per meal.

These guidelines are just that, guidelines. They give you a rough idea of the sort of figures to aim for, but they need to be adapted to **you**. For example, if you've had an extremely active day and just smashed through an epic leg workout, then your portion sizes and carbohydrate consumption can be larger than following an inactive day in the office. The important thing is to evaluate your choices in the context of your whole day. Consider what you're eating for your other meals and snacks and try to make a balanced choice which fits in with these, while also accessing a host of macro and micronutrients.

Beware of the marketing techniques used by high-street stores, cafés and supermarkets. They know that you want to make healthy choices, so will try to sell the supposed health benefits of their meals. Labels that claim food is 'low fat', 'all natural' or 'made with real fruit' should not be mistaken for proof that the food is healthy. These foods can still be poor quality, high in calories and low in nutrients. Be sure to thoroughly read the label before you make your choice.

Labels only tell you so much. They won't tell you about the quality of the ingredients, and how truly natural or fresh they are. These are factors you need to evaluate yourself. As much as the grams of protein, fat or fibre might inform your decision, you also need to consider food quality. For example, the NHS recommend eating no more than 30g of sugar per day, yet a medium apple contains 19g, while a small Milky Bar has 6.9g. I am not going to choose the chocolate over the apple simply because of the sugar content, and neither should you. Take these guidelines with a hefty pinch of salt. Read food labels and combine this information with your knowledge of wholesome foods and micronutrients, as well as your common sense.

And if all else fails... *make a packed lunch!*

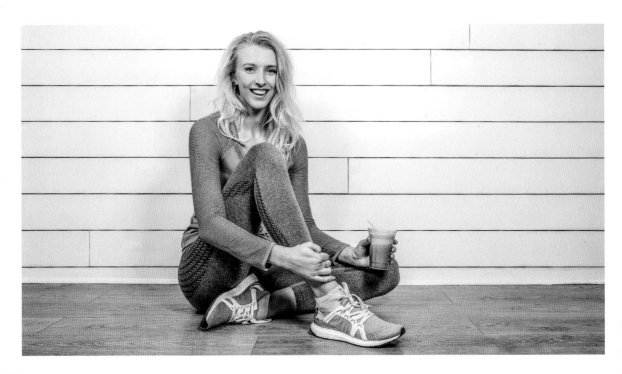

"The best project you'll ever work on is you."

DON'T SWEAT THE SMALL STUFF

I often find that my clients become obsessed with the tiny details. They swear that not eating carbs after 6pm, having 6 small meals a day or consuming only eggs for breakfast is the secret to success. In reality, these tiny details will not massively affect your results. Contrary to popular belief, eating little and often will not burn more fat, and the effect on your metabolic rate is negligible. Your body does not become a fat-storing machine on the stroke of 6pm meaning everything you eat automatically becomes flab. These are myths. What really matters is what you're eating throughout the whole day. What really matters is how often you train and how hard you push yourself. What really matters is that you're making *consistent healthy choices* and *positive changes* to your life, and sticking with them for the long term.

There are no shortcuts when it comes to health. You have to be doing it for the right reasons and you have to stick with it. **Consistency is key.** Instead of focusing on your meal timing and frequency, look at what is in those meals. Instead of concentrating on how many minutes of cardio you're doing, look at whether your workout is challenging your body. It is the overall lifestyle change that

Handling holidays

One of the questions I am asked most frequently is how to handle holidays and weekends away. At times like these, the food available is often out of our control, and we have to eat at restaurants for every single meal. Here are my top tips to stay on track:

- **Try to stay as active as possible.** That doesn't mean go to the gym or do a HIIT workout — unless you really fancy it! You can just explore the local area on foot, go for a hike, swim in the sea or even run up the nearest hill. Just be sure to pack some workout gear so you can get sweaty in style.

- **Take advantage of the local produce.** For example, in hot countries they often serve the most amazing fresh fruit salads, which are perfect for snacking on or sharing with friends. Scout out a local supermarket too, and pick up some healthy snacks such as nuts.

- **Pack wisely.** Travelling can often leave you in a pinch with a rumbling stomach and very few healthy options available. That's why I like to pack a selection of healthy snacks such as home-made trail mix or energy balls. I also like to make sure I've got some natural protein powders with me ready to mix into yoghurt or add to water for a quick protein fix.

- **Do your research.** Before you go away, have a look online for healthy cafés and restaurants. You will be surprised by how many nutritious eateries are popping up all over the world.

will give you the results you want, not the tiny details many get hung up on.

Similarly, don't worry about the occasional slip up. Especially at the beginning of your journey, it can be hard to stick to your new healthy lifestyle. You can find yourself struggling to maintain a balanced diet, or to get to the gym as regularly as you may like. Everyone makes mistakes and *accidentally* drinks a few too many glasses of wine or *somehow* indulges in a few too many slices of pizza. It isn't the end of the world, just be honest with yourself and avoid making excuses for any poor choices. What matters is how you come back from these slip-ups.

If you've had an indulgent day or two and want to get back on track then it helps to avoid the 'dieting mindset' of restriction and deprivation. Instead, reread these balance principles and apply them to your life. Eat delicious, healthy and nutritious foods in abundance. Focus on accessing a range of macro- and micronutrients, colours and natural ingredients. Establish the 80/20 rule and allow yourself to enjoy your favourite treats in moderation. Don't wait for Monday, get back on track right now. Do the best you can and constantly try to improve yourself and your health.

• **Eat consciously.** It is tempting when you're travelling to throw your healthy eating habits out the window. Remember to look after your body. Instead of eating everything in sight, I suggest being mindful of your eating. If you're spending all day laying on a sun lounger, you probably don't need to be eating as much as someone on a hiking holiday. Adapt your portion sizes according to your activity levels. Make the healthiest choices you can at your main meals, applying the balance principles as much as possible. Focus on lean protein, complex carbohydrates, healthy fats and lots of greens. Use my tips for eating at restaurants on pages 153 and 154, but don't be afraid to have a few indulgences. You are on holiday after all!

• **Relax.** The reason you train hard and eat well the vast majority of the time is so you can enjoy these special occasions stress–free. Don't put pressure on yourself to be perfect. Think about it this way: a typical holiday is one week long. That is one week out of your whole year, a week out of your whole *life*. If you smash your health and fitness goals the rest of the time, having a more relaxed approach during a week–long holiday is not the end of the world. It is not going ruin all your progress. It will in fact allow you to relax, de–stress, probably get some vitamin D (depending on the type of holiday you choose) and restore a different kind of balance to your life.

KEEP A HEALTHY MINDSET

Sure, having a healthy body is important but you need a healthy mind too. A key part of a balanced lifestyle is maintaining a relaxed relationship with food and fitness, avoiding obsession, restriction and excessive worrying. So many people who start out on their fitness journey end up taking it too far and developing an unhealthy relationship with training and nutrition in their attempt to get healthy. This can lead to extreme under-eating, over-training, bingeing and feelings of guilt, resulting in a vicious circle that negatively affects not just your physical health, but your mental health too.

I want you to be able to listen to your body, fuel yourself appropriately, train because you love it and accept yourself every step of the way; no guilt, no stress, no restriction and no obsession.

How to maintain a positive relationship with food:

• The first step is to identify your current mindset. It's time to be brutally honest with yourself. Sit back and reflect on your relationship with food. Do you think about it obsessively? Do you feel guilty about eating? Do you train in excess to 'burn off' food? Do you cancel social plans because you want to control your diet? Do you binge? Do you restrict? Focusing on these habits can be an uncomfortable thing to do, but it is absolutely essential.

• Try to avoid the 'dieting' mindset that has been engrained in us from a young age. Instead of seeing healthy eating as a way to lose weight, see it as a positive change to benefit your health and happiness. Instead of seeing exercise as a way to burn off food and fat, see it as a way to strengthen your body and make it fitter and faster. The more you educate yourself about fitness and nutrition the better. Health is about so much more than how you look – it is about how you feel, function and perform. Don't forget that.

• Respect your body. Your body is amazing. It allows you to move, breathe, think, write, speak and love. It is constantly working hard to allow you to *live*. Don't take it for granted. Don't torture it through a restrictive diet and excessive exercise. Instead nourish it with nutrient-dense foods, fuel it with energy and strengthen it with training. Show it the love it shows you.

• Listen to your body. We are inundated with claims about how we should eat, whether it's advice to eat 3, 4, 5 or even 6 times a day, have big breakfasts or always finish the food on our plate. Throw these rules out of the window and don't be afraid to break social norms and routines. Instead, listen to your body. Eat when you're hungry and stop when you're full. If you're craving something sweet, think about what it is that your body **needs**. It's probably not a king-size chocolate bar, but if it is then don't deprive yourself of a few pieces – just make sure you stop when you're satisfied.

• No more 'all or nothing' attitude. People often find that they'll eat a less balanced breakfast and then think 'sod it', and spend the whole day eating poorly. It is essential to avoid this mindset as it can lead to a negative cycle of bingeing and restricting. A key way to do this is to stop labelling foods as good or bad. As soon as we tell ourselves we can't have something, it is all we want. Instead, allow yourself to eat a little bit of everything. See foods as those you eat in abundance, and those you eat in moderation. That way, nothing is out of bounds and no guilt is attached to any food.

• If you do binge, take a step back and reflect on why you did so. Grab a pen and paper and write down how it made you feel, and read this next time you feel the urge to overeat. Seek out activities you enjoy and can use as a distraction when you feel the urge to binge, such as calling a friend or going for a walk. Ultimately binge eating is a habit, a habit that you can break with hard work, determination and self-belief, so stick with it.

• If you find that you struggle to maintain self-control with certain food, then remove it from your vicinity or buy portion-controlled packs. For example, I can easily overeat on nut butter, so I buy individual serving-sized sachets to avoid grabbing a teaspoon and working my way through a whole jar!

• If you do overeat or just go out for a big meal with friends or family, do not weigh yourself the following morning. It is likely that you will gain a lot of 'water weight' as when you eat more salty food, as social and celebratory foods often are, it causes your body to retain water in its cells. Do not confuse this with actual weight gain. Stepping on the scales can encourage feelings of guilt and make you want you restrict your diet or exercise excessively to 'balance out' what you ate the day before. Doing this only fuels the negative cycle of bingeing and restricting, so try to avoid it.

• There is much more to life than food and fitness. **So. Much. More.** It can be easy to fall in love with healthy living and take it to a point of obsession without even realising it. If you find that it is interfering with your social life or relationships, it is time to take a step back and reflect. Training and nutrition are not the be all and end all. Sure, they are pretty damn important when it comes to maintaining good health and looking after yourself, but they shouldn't significantly hinder other positive elements of your life. Sometimes work, family or life in general has to come first, and that's okay. Health and fitness should be part of your life, but don't let it become your whole life.

• Acknowledge that failure is normal and to be expected. You can't miraculously turn into a perfectly healthy, fit and balanced person overnight. There will be times when you overeat or undereat, times when you train too much or too little, and times when you doubt yourself and your abilities. That's okay. What matters is that you avoid feelings of guilt and just try to get back on track as soon as you can. Stay positive and remind yourself *why* you're making these healthy choices.

Note: These are my personal tips and tricks to maintaining a healthy and a balanced relationship with food. If you're really struggling or feel like you may be developing a disordered relationship with food, seek professional help.

FEEL THE SELF-LOVE

People often hear the phrase 'self-love' and cringe. I want to change that. Self-love is a huge part of a healthy mindset. How can you expect to care for your body and maintain a positive relationship with food and fitness when you have a negative relationship with yourself?

When people see my transformation pictures, they see only the physical changes; what they don't notice are the mental ones. I have been through a long process of self-acceptance. I've gone from focusing on my flaws and never being satisfied with my progress, to completely and utterly loving, not only my body, but my mind, and accepting myself for who I really am – which is so much more than how I look.

Loving yourself is a choice. A choice that **you** can make. Admittedly, it is a challenge. Especially in a world where we are conditioned to pull ourselves apart. Multi-million pound industries rely on us being self-critical and play on our insecurities. Images of perfection, many of which are digitally manipulated, are thrust in our faces at every turn. It is not encouraged to be confident or happy in yourself. We are all eager to be self-deprecating, pessimistic or negative. In a society like this, we can't be blamed for doubting ourselves.

We need to open ourselves up to the possibility of body-positivity. In reality, if you do not accept your body at the beginning of your fitness journey, you will never be satisfied. You need to love yourself first. Before anything else. Before you lose weight. Before you get fit. Before you get your 'dream body'. If you tell yourself, 'I'll be happy with myself once I am a size 10' or 'once I have abs', you will never be satisfied. Once

you achieve one goal you will find something else you have to do before you can be happy. This leads to a vicious circle of never being truly satisfied with yourself, your body or your life. You need to allow yourself to love yourself and be happy right here, right now. This will allow you to embark on your fitness journey for the right reasons, not from a place of self-hate but from a place of self-love. You will make positive and lasting changes because you *love* your body and want to take care of it.

It's all very well telling you to love yourself, but how do you actually do that? It's tough and it takes time, but it is possible. Here are my top tips to get started:

• Reflect on your relationship with yourself. Is it a good one? Are you happy in who you are a person? Do you feel limited by your own lack of self-belief? Do you want to love yourself more? You have to actively choose to think more positively and to make a change to your mindset. Don't get me wrong here, self-love isn't about thinking you're the badger's nadgers. It is just about accepting yourself, warts and all, and working on being the best version of you.

• Reflect on who you are as a person, beyond how you look. What really makes you **you**? Think about your best friend. Why do you love them? I'm pretty certain it is because of their kindness, sense of humour or intelligence, not their thigh gap. People love you because of who you are, not because of your appearance. Place value on your personality rather than your appearance, and self-love becomes a whole lot more achievable.

• Surround yourself with positive and empowering people. The sort of people who bring you up, compliment you, encourage you and make you feel amazing. Try to remove negative people from your life, or at the very least spend less time with them. If you're struggling to find others on your wavelength then don't be afraid to meet new people through social events, new hobbies or even online.

• Comparison is the thief of joy. We are constantly bombarded with images of other people with perfect bodies, perfect relationships and perfect lives. We compare ourselves and end up feeling like we don't live up to the standards everyone else is setting. The reality is, those standards don't exist. The people you see in the mainstream media or on social media are airbrushed, edited, filtered and Photoshopped to portray an image of perfection. Beyond appearances, they often share only the best bits of their lives. The happy moments and the highlights. And you know what? That's okay. That is the nature of the media. What matters is that you don't absorb this content, assume it is real and then compare yourself to it. See it for what it is – a false representation of reality. Take inspiration and motivation, but do not compare.

• Love your imperfections. No one, **and I mean no one**, is perfect. Every single person has flaws. Every single person has down days, slips up, fails and is rejected. Every person cries. Your flaws do not define who you are. What really matters is how you respond to them. Even if you can't love them, at least try to accept them and then go from there. We are perfectly imperfect.

• Think about all the time you have spent worrying about how you look or what other people think about you. Now imagine if you had spent that time on something positive

like building your career or bonding with your loved ones. All of a sudden picking yourself apart seems like a big waste of time, doesn't it? We aren't here forever, so use your time and energy wisely.

• On a similar note, realise the value of self-love. It manifests as self-belief, and with self-belief you are extremely powerful. You are confident in who you are and your abilities, and you can do anything you set your mind to. You develop qualities such as grit, the ability to get back up after rejection of failure; and you become comfortable with going out of your comfort zone to achieve your goals. And, ultimately, these skills will help you achieve success in all areas of your life.

• Work on being positive in all aspects of your life, beyond body image. Try to see the good in every situation and don't waste your energy on moaning, complaining or getting angry about small things. Spread happiness by bringing up others, complimenting them and encouraging them. Be the kind of person you want to meet. At the end of each day I like to do a quick self-development task that takes only minutes. I ask myself what were three positive things that happened in the day, and one way in which I could improve the next day. This enables you to find the good in every single day, even the really rubbish ones, and also lets you reflect on yourself and your actions.

• Talk to yourself... yep, really. This is where it starts to get a bit cheesy, but I promise this works. Take time each day to look in the mirror and point out three things you love about yourself. Not just your body, but who you are as a person. Tell yourself that you love yourself, that you love your body and that you're going to take care of it. This is especially effective if you do it in the morning, as it sets you up with a positive mindset for the day ahead and motivates you to make healthy and happy choices throughout the day.

• Realise that it is perfectly okay to love yourself. No one is going to think you're arrogant. If anyone ever says something negative about you, it is a direct reflection of their own lack of self-worth. People who are happy in themselves do not criticise and bring down others. Break the mould of self-deprecation. Smile at strangers, walk with a spring in your step and let your positivity light up a room.

A BALANCED APPROACH TO FOOD

So that's it, my nutrition principles, which you can apply to your life to achieve lasting health and happiness. I know that 'balance' can seem elusive, but it is much simpler than you think. Balance is about consistently making the best choices you can and fuelling yourself with nutritious foods that make you feel energised. It is not about cutting out food groups, detoxing or depriving yourself of your favourite treats. It is about awareness of what you're putting into your body, making small changes towards a healthier you and enjoying delicious food that is full of flavour along the way.

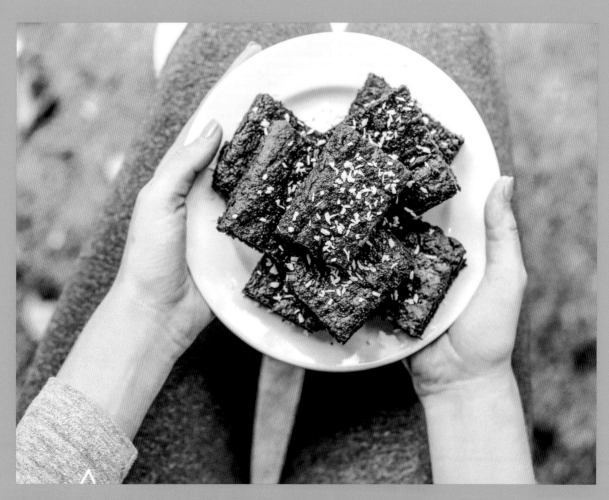

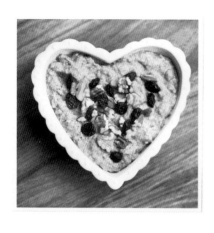
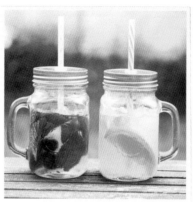
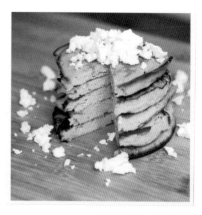

THE RECIPES

Now for the fun stuff. Let's get cooking!

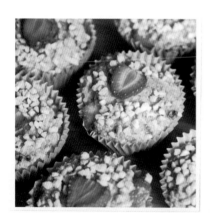
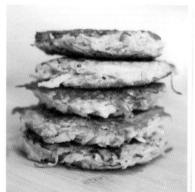
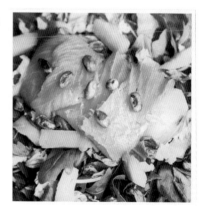

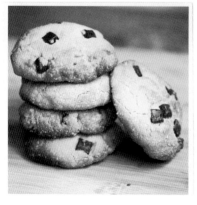
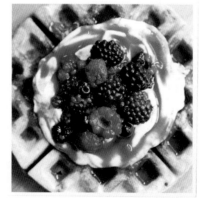
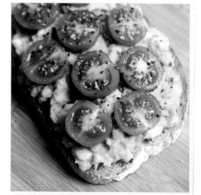

The recipes that follow are designed to be quick, simple and delicious. They don't require any funky ingredients and they're crammed full of flavour. Many of them can be packed up and taken to work, perfect for when you're making your own lunchbox. In terms of portion sizes, feel free to adapt these to your needs.

I recommend preparing food in advance if you're often on the go. The vast majority of these meals last well in airtight containers stored in the fridge and you can freeze them to make them stay fresh even longer. Try doubling up a meal and saving the extra for lunch the next day. You can even bulk-make a recipe and spread it throughout the week. Not only will this save you money but it also helps you stay on track with your healthy lifestyle and avoid the temptation of the office canteen.

Just a couple of things I want to touch on before you head to the kitchen are:

- **Oils for cooking.**
When it comes to cold dishes such as salads I like to drizzle over olive oil. I tend to stick with coconut oil when heating foods to high temperatures as it is one of the most stable oils under these conditions. I know that coconut oil can seem expensive at first but the price is slowly coming down and you only use a tiny amount so it is great value for money. Trust me, it's worth it!

- **Oven temperatures.**
All oven temperatures are for fan ovens, unless otherwise stated.

- **Eggs.**
All eggs in the recipes are medium size and free-range. I like to source mine locally.

- **Milk.**
When I use milk in a recipe, I use either a variety of cow's milk or a non-dairy alternative such as coconut, soya or almond milk.

Brace yourself, you're about to see some serious food porn.

BREAKFAST

LEMON AND COCONUT OVERNIGHT OATS

This is one of my favourite breakfast recipes for the warmer months and it's super-simple. Just pop all the ingredients in a container and chill overnight, then you can grab and go in the morning.

SERVES 1

50g (2oz) porridge oats
20g (¾oz) unsweetened
   desiccated coconut
70g (2¼oz) natural Greek
   yoghurt
½ tsp vanilla extract
1 tbsp honey or maple syrup
grated zest of 1 unwaxed
   lemon
1 tbsp chia seeds (optional)
150ml (5fl oz) milk
toppings of your choice
   (e.g. fresh berries or chopped
   nuts), to serve

1. Combine the oats and coconut in a bowl, then add the yoghurt, vanilla extract, honey or maple syrup and lemon zest and stir thoroughly until combined.

If you're using chia seeds add them with all the milk, however if you're not using them just add 100ml (3½fl oz) of the milk and be aware that the finished oats won't be as creamy.

2. Transfer the mixture to a container, seal with a lid and pop it in the fridge. Leave it overnight to thicken up and add toppings of your choice in the morning (I love fresh blueberries).

Tip: You can add protein powder to the mixture before leaving it to soak overnight but, depending on the type of powder you use, you will need to add more liquid to compensate for the drying nature of the powder.

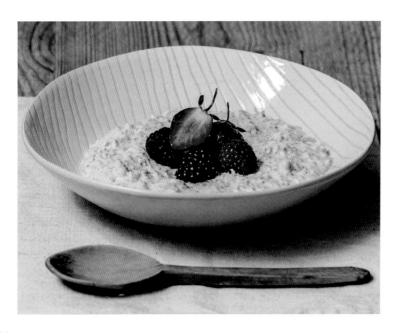

CINNAMON SPICE PROTEIN ZOATS

The concept of courgette in oats baffles a lot of people, however I pinky promise that you can't taste it; it just gives you a larger volume of food and a serving of greens: winner winner!

SERVES 1

½—⅔ medium courgette
50g (2oz) porridge oats
½ tsp ground cinnamon
½ tsp ground allspice
1 tbsp natural sweetener
  e.g. stevia or honey
150ml (5fl oz) milk or water
1 scoop (25g/1oz) protein
  powder
toppings of your choice
  (I like 1 tbsp raisins, 1 tbsp
  walnuts, 1 tbsp pecans),
  to serve

1. Grate the courgette and combine it with the oats, cinnamon, allspice, sweetener and milk or water in a microwave-safe bowl.

2. Pop the bowl in a microwave and cook on high for 1½-2 minutes, or until almost all the liquid has been absorbed. Alternatively, cook the courgette mixture in a pan over a medium heat on the hob for 3-5 minutes, until the liquid has almost all been absorbed.

3. Remove from the microwave of from the hob and stir through the protein powder, then leave the mixture to sit for a minute and thicken up.

4. Add toppings of your choice and serve.

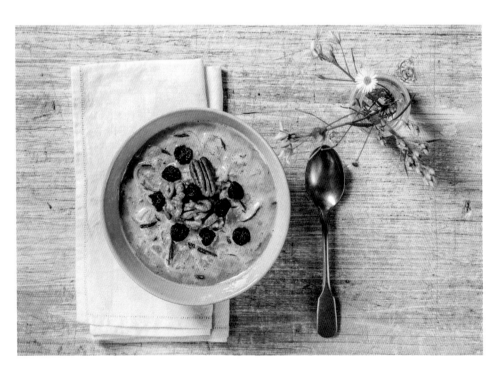

BERRY MINT SMOOTHIE

This fresh flavoursome smoothie is packed full of micronutrients and is the perfect way to start your day.

SERVES 1

2 tbsp natural Greek yoghurt
handful of spinach leaves
6—8 mint leaves
1 large banana, frozen
60g (2oz) frozen raspberries
   or mixed berries
5 ice cubes
250ml (9fl oz) milk

1.   Place all the ingredients in a blender or food processor and blitz until smooth. You might need to stir the mixture or shake the blender to help all the ingredients combine. The end result is a thick, creamy and delicious milkshake that is packed full of flavour.

Tip: You can add a scoop of protein powder to this shake but will need to add an extra 50ml (2fl oz) liquid if you do so.

Tip: When freezing bananas, I recommend leaving them to ripen until they're pretty brown. Then peel them and pop them in the freezer, to produce the sweetest, most delicious shakes.

NUTTY GREEN MILKSHAKE

This super-simple green milkshake tastes like banana peanut butter heaven, with hidden goodness! I like to use unsweetened almond milk in my shakes as it is low in calories and adds a sweet, nutty flavour.

SERVES 1

1 large banana, frozen
10 ice cubes
1 heaped tbsp natural
   peanut butter
handful of spinach leaves
225ml (8fl oz) milk

1.   Place all the ingredients in a blender or food processor and blitz until smooth. You might need to stir the mixture or shake the blender to help all the ingredients combine. I promise it's worth it, as the end product is super thick and creamy, just like a milkshake!

Tip: You can add a scoop of protein powder to this shake but you will need to add an extra 50ml (2fl oz) liquid if you do so.

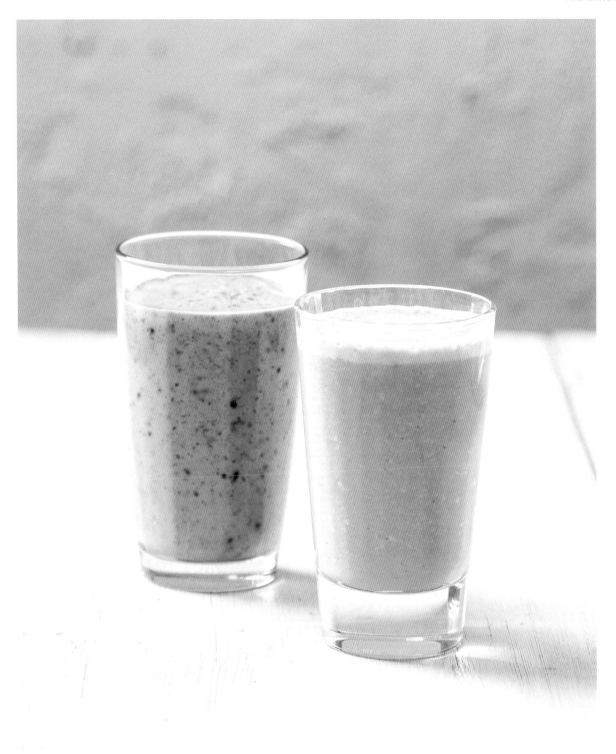

TOAST TOPPINGS

Toast doesn't have to be boring. There are so many delicious and balanced ways that you can top a humble slice of bread, and here are my favourites.

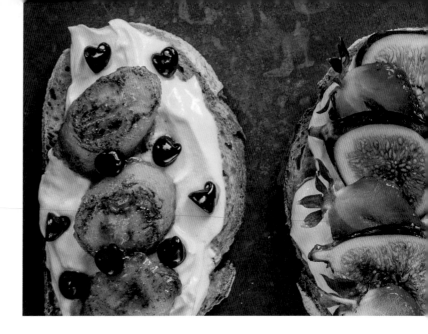

Sweet

HONEY, RICOTTA, LEMON AND SLICED FRUIT
SERVES 1

2 heaped tbsp ricotta cheese
juice of ½ lemon
½ tbsp honey
fruit of your choice (strawberries
   and figs work best)
1 slice of bread

1. Combine the ricotta, lemon juice and honey in a bowl and set aside.

2. Finely slice the fruit.

3. Toast the bread and spread it with a layer of the ricotta mixture, then top with the sliced fruit. Bosh!

Sweet

GREEK YOGHURT, CARAMELISED BANANA AND DARK CHOCOLATE CHIPS
SERVES 1

1 tsp coconut oil
½ banana, thickly sliced
1 tsp ground cinnamon
1 tsp honey or natural sweetener
1 slice of bread
2 tbsp natural Greek yoghurt
1 tbsp dark chocolate chips
   or chopped dark chocolate
   (70% cocoa solids)

1. Heat the coconut oil in a pan over a medium heat add the slices of banana. Fry lightly for 1 minute, until the banana slices are golden brown on the underside, then sprinkle over half the cinnamon and drizzle over half the honey or sweetener and flip the slices. Add the remaining honey or sweetener and cinnamon and fry until brown on the other side. Remove from the heat and leave to cool while you toast the bread.

2. Toast the bread, spread with the yoghurt, top with a layer of fried banana slices and scatter with the chocolate chips or broken chocolate.

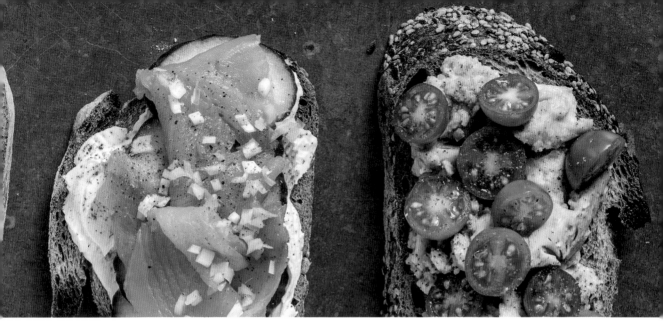

Savoury

SMOKED SALMON, CUCUMBER AND CREAM CHEESE

SERVES 1

1 slice of bread
1 heaped tbsp cream cheese
6 cucumber slices
50g (2oz) smoked salmon
1 spring onion, finely chopped
black pepper

1. Toast the bread and spread it with the cream cheese.

2. Lay the cucumber slices over the cheese, followed by the salmon. Finally, sprinkle over the spring onion and grind over some black pepper to taste.

Savoury

MASHED AVOCADO AND CHERRY TOMATOES

SERVES 1

½ ripe avocado
pinch of salt
1 slice of bread
5 cherry tomatoes, halved
black pepper

1. Scoop out the avocado flesh and mash it in a bowl with the salt using a fork.

2. Toast the bread and top it with the mashed avocado and cherry tomatoes. Grind over some black pepper to taste.

SWEET POTATO PANCAKES

These two-ingredient sweet potato pancakes are ridiculously easy to make and provide a versatile and delicious base for a whole host of toppings.

SERVES 1

1 small sweet potato
2 medium eggs
1 tsp coconut oil
toppings of your choice,
    such as feta, poached eggs,
    or yoghurt and fruit, to serve

1. Pierce the sweet potato and place it in the microwave, then cook on High for 5-7 minutes, until cooked through (alternatively, pierce and bake in the oven until tender). Leave for a few minutes until cool enough to handle, then remove the flesh.

2. Add 150g (5oz) of the sweet potato flesh to a blender with the eggs and blitz to form a smooth batter.

3. Heat the coconut oil in a non-stick frying pan over a low-medium heat and pop a 5cm-wide dollop of batter in the centre. Fry gently for 30-60 seconds until the base is firm, then flip with a spatula and continue frying for a further 30-60 seconds until cook through and golden brown. Remove from the heat, then repeat with the remaining batter to produce 5-6 pancakes and serve with toppings of your choice.

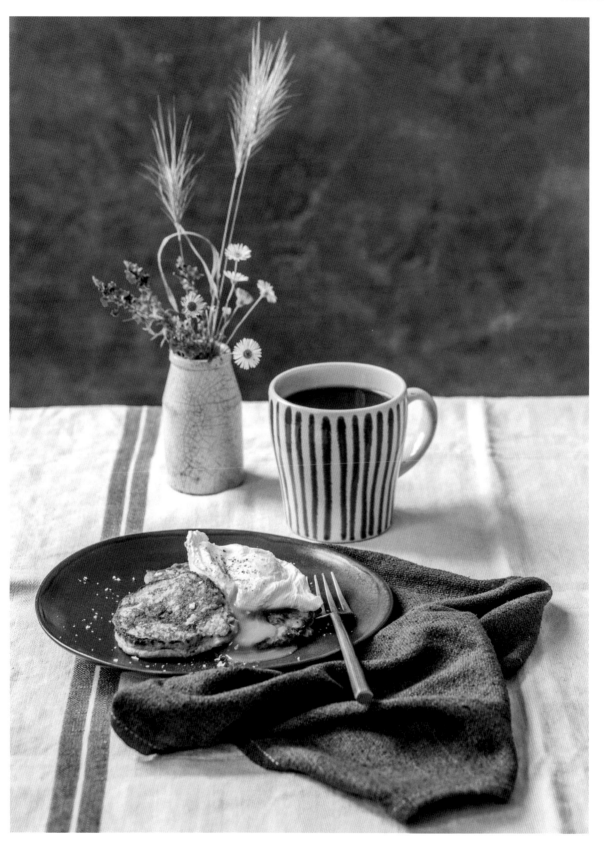

CHEESY COURGETTE FRITTERS WITH YOGHURT AND CHIVE DIP

These fritters are a great way to get your greens in at breakfast, plus they're insanely moreish!

SERVES 1—2 (DEPENDING ON HOW HUNGRY YOU ARE)

For the fritters
2 medium courgettes
   (250—300g/9—10½oz),
   grated
2 large eggs, lightly beaten
25g (1oz) grated Parmesan
20g (¾oz) ground almond flour
   (or plain flour)
salt and black pepper
coconut oil, for frying

For the yoghurt and chive dip
3 tbsp natural full-fat Greek
   yoghurt
juice of ½ lemon
1 medium garlic clove, minced
1 tbsp finely snipped fresh chives
pinch of salt
1 tsp olive oil

1. To make the yoghurt and chive dip, simply combine the ingredients in a small bowl, then set aside.

2. Place the grated courgettes in a clean tea towel, then squeeze over the sink to get rid of as much excess liquid as possible (trust me, you need to make sure the courgette is dry!).

3. Transfer the grated courgette to a bowl and add the eggs, grated Parmesan and flour, then season with salt and pepper.

4. Heat a little coconut oil in a non-stick pan over a low-medium heat. Grab a small handful of the batter and form into a patty. Place in the pan and fry for 3-4 minutes until golden brown on the bottom, then flip and fry on the other side for 1-2 minutes, or until cooked through. Repeat with the remaining batter (you'll end up with about 4 fritters), adding more coconut oil if needed, then serve the fritters warm with the dip.

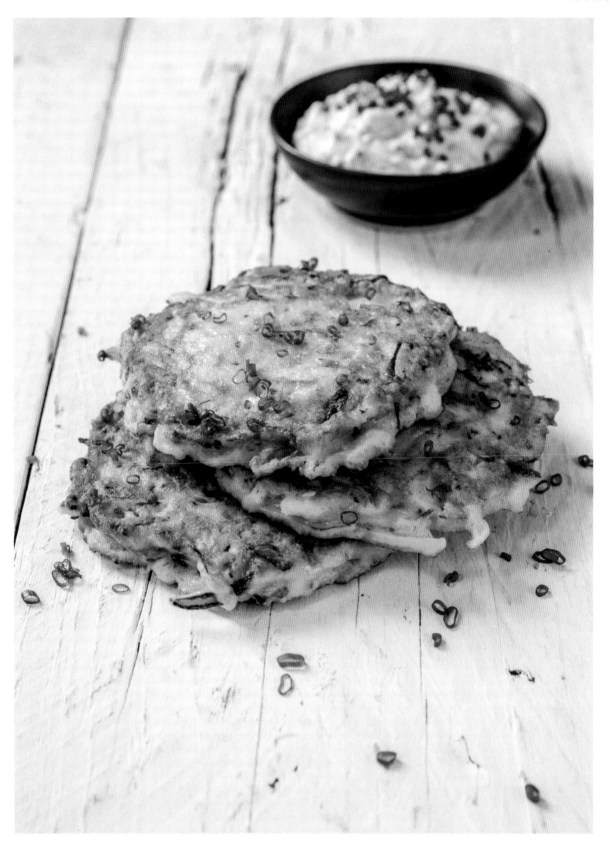

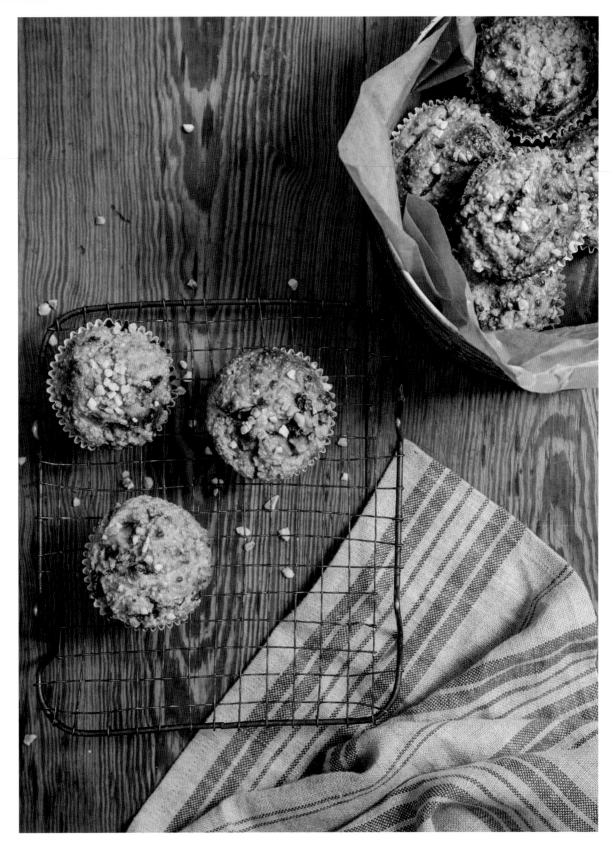

STRAWBERRY SHORTCAKE BREAKFAST MUFFINS

These scrummy muffins can be baked in advance and then grabbed in the morning as a quick and easy on-the-go breakfast.

MAKES 6—8 MUFFINS

200g (7oz) porridge oats
2 eggs, lightly beaten
150g (5oz) natural full–fat
  Greek yoghurt
50ml (2fl oz) milk
50g (2oz) clear honey
½ tsp baking powder
½ tsp bicarbonate of soda
125g (4½oz) hulled and roughly
  chopped strawberries
3—4 tbsp chopped almonds
  (optional)

1. Preheat the oven to 180°C/350°F/Gas Mk 4 and line a 12-hole muffin tray with 6-8 muffin cases.

2. Blitz the oats in a blender or food processor until a fine flour is formed. Tip the oat flour into a bowl and add the eggs, yoghurt, milk, honey, baking powder and bicarbonate of soda and mix until combined (do not over-mix). Add the strawberries and gently stir them through, retaining some for garnishing the finished muffins, if you wish.

3. Spoon the batter into the muffin cases, and sprinkle with chopped almonds for added crunch (if using). Bake for about 15 minutes (20 minutes if making 6 larger muffins), until cooked through, golden and just firm to the touch, then remove from the oven and leave to cool in the tin.

Tip: Use silicone or foil muffin cases, as these muffins don't fare well with paper ones, unless they're non–stick. Alternatively, try scrunching up some squares of baking parchment then smoothing them out and using them to line the tray instead of cases.

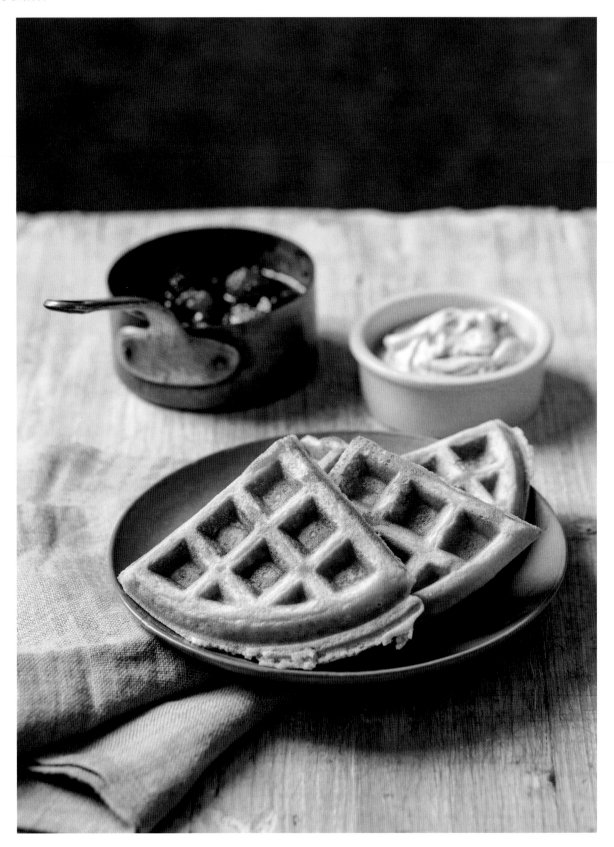

PROTEIN WAFFLE WITH CINNAMON GREEK YOGHURT AND WARM BERRIES

This waffle is high in protein and packed full of flavour, providing the perfect balanced breakfast to kick-start your day. If you don't have a waffle iron, the mixture works perfectly as a pancake batter, cooked in a regular frying pan.

SERVES 1 (MAKES 1 WAFFLE OR ABOUT 4 PANCAKES)

75g (2½oz) frozen berries
cooking spray or coconut oil

For the waffle
25g (1oz) porridge oats
one scoop (25g/1oz) protein
  powder
1 medium egg
3 tbsp milk
1 tbsp maple syrup
½ tsp vanilla extract
¼ tsp baking powder

For the cinnamon yoghurt
100g (3½oz) natural Greek
  yoghurt (full–fat or 0% fat)
½ tsp ground cinnamon
1 tsp clear honey

1. To make the yoghurt, mix together all the ingredients in a bowl. Set aside.

2. For the waffle, start by blitzing the oats in a blender or food processor until a flour is formed. Add the remaining ingredients and blitz again to form a smooth batter, scraping down the sides and adding a splash more milk if needed, to make a batter the consistency of thick double cream.

3. Spray the waffle maker (if using) with cooking spray and pour in the batter, spreading it evenly across the plates. Cook for about 3 minutes, or according to the manufacturer's instructions. For pancakes, melt a little coconut oil in a non-stick frying pan over a medium heat. Add large spoonfuls of the batter to the pan and cook for about 2 minutes, or until small bubbles appear on top and the bottom is golden brown. Flip over and cook for a further 1–2 minutes. Transfer to a plate and repeat with remaining batter, adding more oil if needed. You should be able to cook 2 pancakes at a time, depending on the size of your frying pan.

4. Pop the berries in a microwave-safe bowl and microwave on High for around 1½ minutes, stirring every 30 seconds, until soft and warm. Alternatively, place in a small saucepan over a medium heat, bring to a simmer and cook for 2-3 minutes.

5. Place the waffle or pancakes on the plate, add the yoghurt and berries, devour and enjoy!

SMOKED CAULIFLOWER KEDGEREE

Using cauliflower 'rice' keeps this kedgeree super light and makes it a great low carbohydrate breakfast dish. At first glance this recipe might seem complicated, but it is incredibly quick and easy to make.

SERVES 2

4 eggs
1 large head of cauliflower, broken into florets
coconut oil, for frying
2 garlic cloves, minced
1 tsp freshly grated root ginger
1 tsp curry powder
½ tsp dried chilli flakes (optional)
½ tsp mustard seeds
½ tsp ground turmeric
small handful of coriander, finely chopped
2 small smoked, cooked fish fillets (mackerel or haddock are best), flaked
salt and black pepper

1. First things first, boil the eggs. Pop them in a pan, cover with water, and place over the heat. As soon as the water begins to boil, take the pan off the heat, cover and leave to sit for 9 minutes. Then drain and cool the eggs under cold running water. Remove the shells and set the eggs aside.

2. Make the cauliflower 'rice' by blitzing the florets in a food processor until they resemble grains of rice, or grating them against the holes of a fine grater.

3. Heat a little coconut oil in a non-stick large frying pan and add the cauliflower rice with the garlic. Fry for 5 minutes, stirring, then add the spices, mix them through and cook for a further 5 minutes until the cauliflower is tender. Take off the heat and stir through the fish and fresh coriander. Season to taste.

4. Halve the boiled eggs, pop them on top of the kedgeree, and serve.

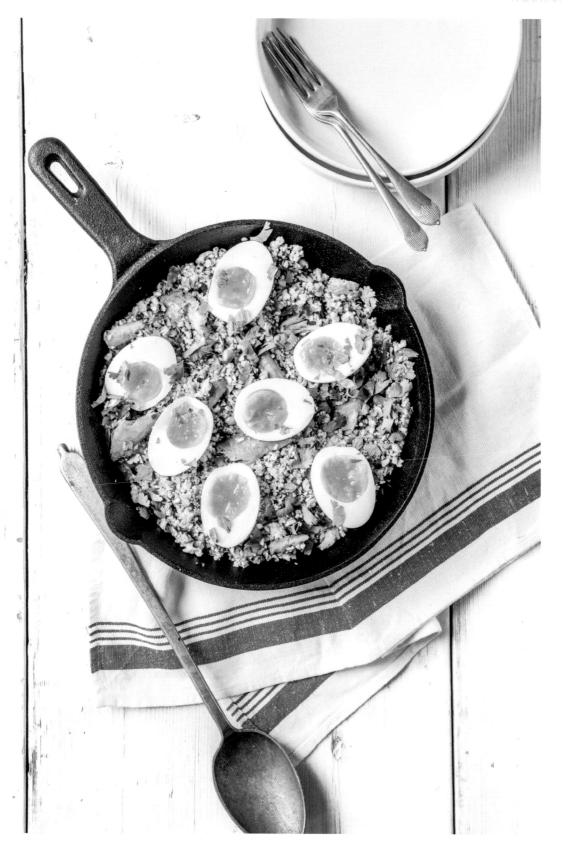

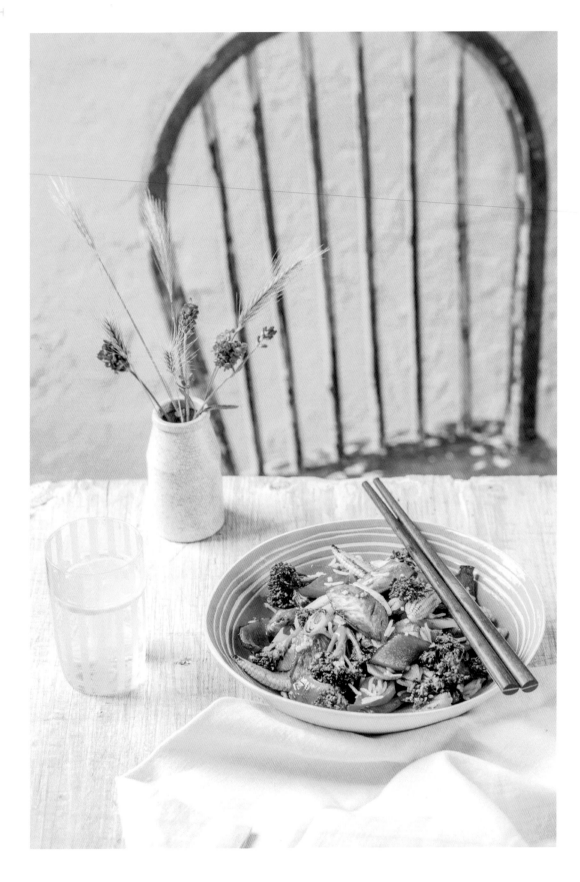

THE BASIC CHICKEN STIR FRY

Stir fries are extremely versatile and easy. You literally just shove everything in a pan over a high heat and cook it through. This recipe is a great starting point – feel free to experiment with other protein sources such as tofu or prawns, as well as veggies and seasonings. Go wild!

MAKES 1 GENEROUS SERVING
OR 2 SMALLER SERVINGS

1 tbsp coconut oil
1 chicken breast, cut into
   bite–sized chunks
prepared vegetables of choice
   (e.g. red onion, peppers,
   baby sweetcorn, Tenderstem
   broccoli), cut into bite–sized
   chunks (about 200—250g/
   7—9oz prepared veg, in total)
1 tbsp freshly grated root ginger
2 tbsp soy sauce
2 tsp sesame oil
rice, to serve

1. Heat the oil in pan over a medium-high heat and fry the chicken until just cooked through, then set aside.

2. Add the veggies to the pan with the ginger and stir-fry for a couple of minutes, then add a couple of tablespoons of water and gently simmer until the water evaporates and the vegetables have softened. Continue frying to crisp them up a little (this keeps the veggies super-juicy), then tip the meat back into the pan along with the soy sauce and sesame oil. Stir-fry for a couple of minutes, then remove from the heat.

3. Serve with rice. I personally like to get a pack of cooked rice and add half of it to the pan a few minutes before the stir fry's ready, so it absorbs the flavours.

SMASHED BUTTER BEAN AND AVOCADO OPEN-FACE SANDWICH

This sandwich is packed full of flavour as well as fibre, to keep you feeling fuller for longer. By making the sandwich open faced you halve the typical bread intake.

SERVES 2—3

1 x 400g tin of butter beans, drained and rinsed
1 ripe avocado, halved, stoned and sliced
juice of ½ lemon
1 heaped tbsp pesto
1 tbsp natural Greek yoghurt
6—8 basil leaves, finely chopped
2—3 large slices of bread
salt and black pepper

1. Pat the beans dry with kitchen paper, put into a bowl and mash to form a paste.

2. Add the avocado and lemon juice to the butter beans and mash until the mixture has a smooth consistency. Stir in the pesto, yoghurt and basil, then season to taste.

3. Dollop the mixture onto the bread slices, spread evenly and devour!

Tip: For a flavour twist, substitute the pesto for a tablespoon of Dijon mustard.

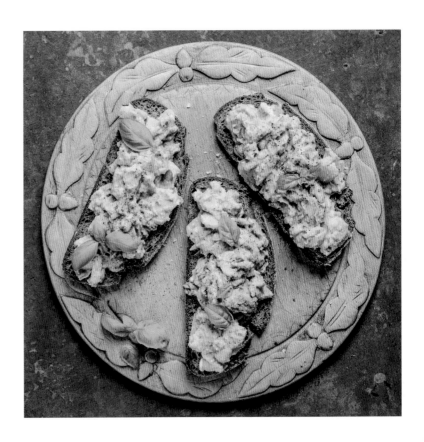

SMOKED SALMON, MANGO AND PISTACHIO SALAD

This salad is inspired by a dish I tried on a trip to Rome, which combined these flavours. Admittedly the ingredients are a little costly but I promise the outcome is worth it. This salad is ideal for special occasions or when you're just feeling fancy. You don't need a dressing as the ingredients are so flavoursome.

SERVES 2

80—100g (2¾—4oz) bag rocket

1 Little Gem lettuce, sliced

120g (4oz) pack of smoked salmon

½ ripe mango (about 150g/5oz), sliced

4 tbsp pistachios

1. Just grab a couple of bowls and divide the ingredients between them. Simples!

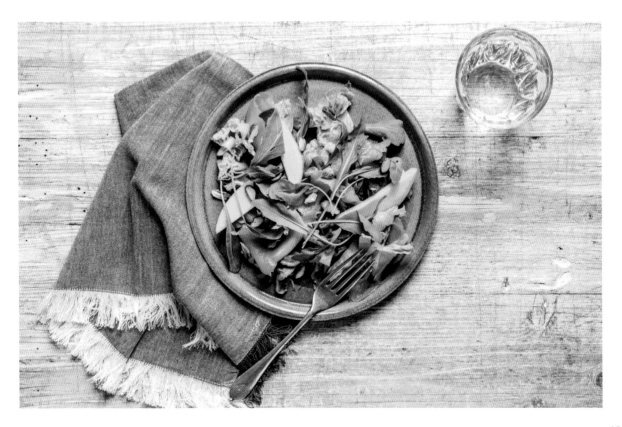

SEARED BEEF AND GARLIC MUSHROOM SALAD

Vegetarians, look away now! This juicy beef salad packs a serious protein hit and is a great light lunch to make ahead of time and pack to eat on the go.

SERVES 2

2 tbsp sesame seeds
2 small steaks of your choice
  (I use rump steak)
coconut oil, for rubbing
  and frying
salt and black pepper
200—250g (7—9oz) button or
  cup mushrooms, quartered
1 large garlic clove, minced
handful of chopped coriander,
  to serve
salad or mixed leaves, to serve

For the dressing
2 tbsp soy sauce
2 tbsp white wine vinegar
1 tsp olive oil
1 tsp freshly grated root ginger

1. Toast the sesame seeds in a dry frying pan over a medium heat until golden brown, then remove from the heat and set aside.

2. Combine the dressing ingredients in a bowl or jar, and set aside.

3. Rub the steaks with oil on each side and sprinkle with salt, pepper and the toasted seeds, pressing the seeds and seasoning into the steak. Set aside.

4. Heat a little coconut oil in a pan over a medium-high heat. Add the mushrooms and garlic and sauté for 7-8 minutes until browned, then transfer to a plate.

5. Add a teaspoon of oil to the pan and fry the steaks 2-4 minutes on each side, depending on how well you like them cooked. Transfer to a board, leave to rest for a minute or two, then slice up.

6. Load up your plate with the salad, the mushrooms and the steak. Sprinkle over the coriander and pour over the dressing. Tuck in!

Tip: I always use rump steaks in this salad as they are cheap yet still full of flavour and easy to cook.

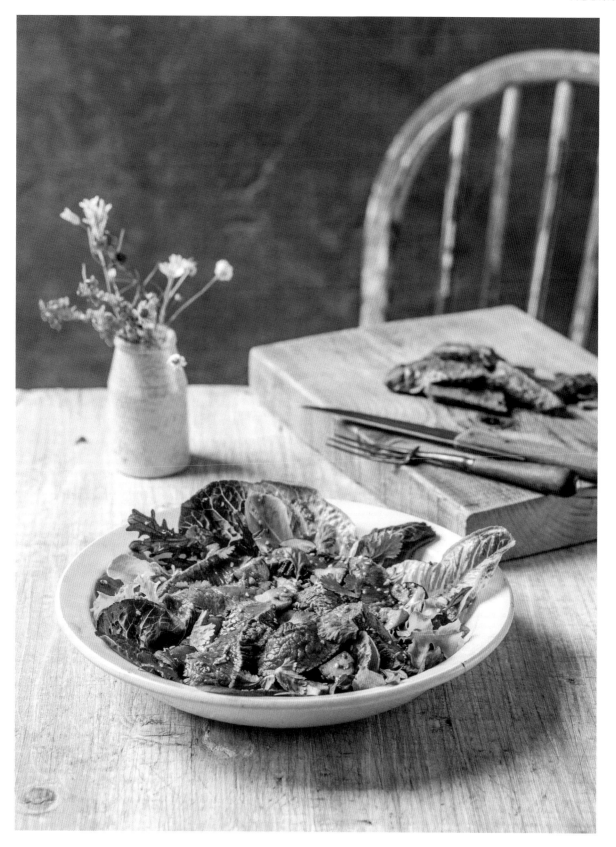

SWEET POTATO AND BLACK BEAN BURRITO
Vegan friendly!

If I could only eat one thing for the rest of my life, it would be burritos. So I just had to share my favourite (vegan-friendly!) burrito recipe.

SERVES 3—4

1 ripe avocado, halved and
   stoned
1 garlic clove, minced
¼ tsp dried chilli flakes
juice of ½ lime
pinch of salt
coconut oil, for frying
1 red onion, diced
½ large red pepper, seeded
   and diced
1 small sweet potato, peeled
   and diced
400g tin of black beans,
   drained and rinsed
1 tsp smoked paprika
½ tsp ground cumin
¼ tsp chilli powder (mild,
   medium or hot depending on
   your preference)
salt and black pepper
3—4 large wholewheat tortillas
1 Little Gem lettuce, shredded

1. Scoop the avocado flesh into a bowl and mash it with the garlic, chilli flakes, lime juice and salt.

2. Heat a little coconut oil in a large frying pan over a medium heat, then add the diced onion, pepper and sweet potato and fry for a couple of minutes until the vegetables soften and brown. Add 100ml (3½fl oz) water, then cover and cook for 8-10 minutes until the sweet potato is soft when pierced with a fork. Add the black beans and spices, then season. Cook, stirring, for a further 3-5 minutes, until the beans are warmed through.

3. Warm the tortillas in the microwave on high for 15 seconds, or in a warm oven for a minute or two. Serve by stuffing each wrap with some of the lettuce, sweet potato and bean mixture, and mashed avocado.

Tip: Meat eaters can of course add a protein source of their choice to this recipe. Chicken chunks, or strips of pork or beef work well.

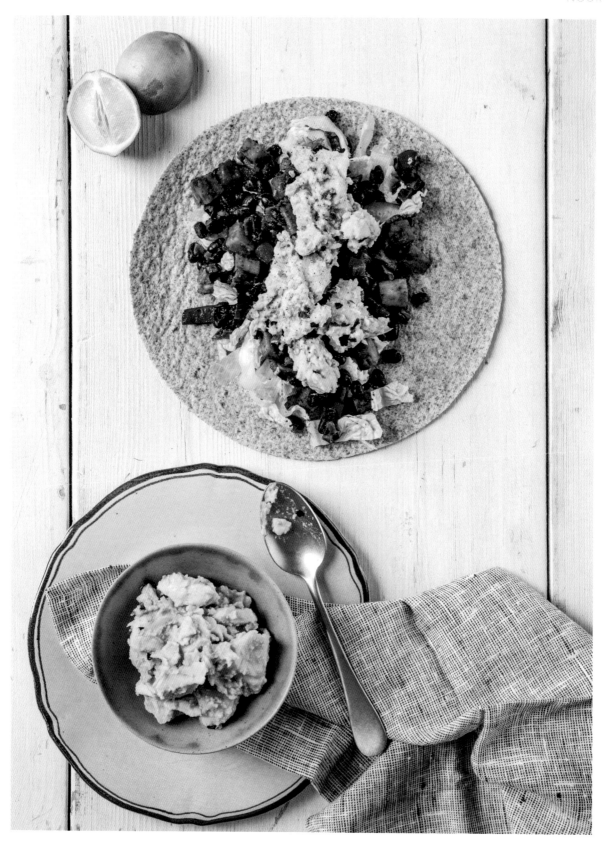

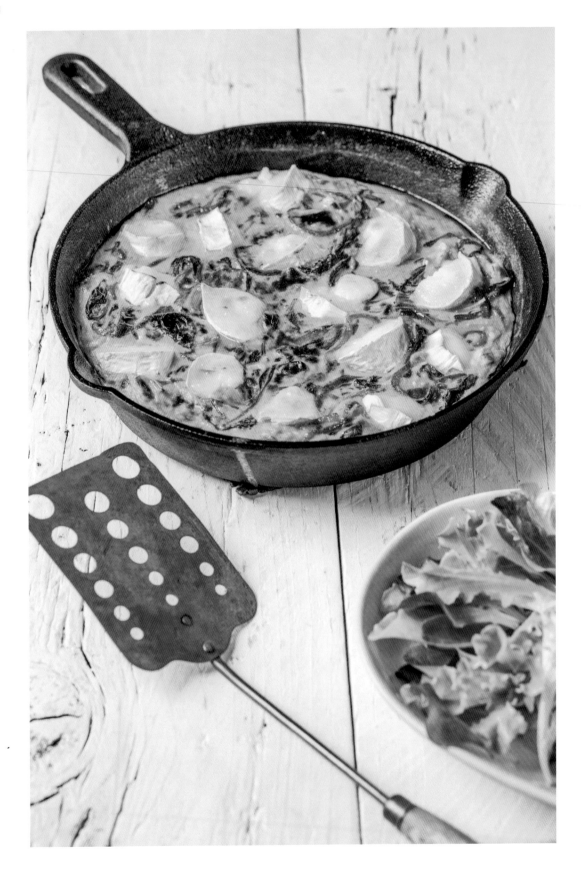

CARAMELISED ONION, SPINACH AND GOATS' CHEESE FRITTATA

This is my favourite lunch recipe in the book. It's extremely easy to make, yet tastes absolutely incredi. Plus, it stores well in a sealed Tupperware box, making a perfect on-the-go lunch.

SERVES 3

8 large free–range eggs
50ml (2fl oz) milk
2 tsp coconut oil
2 large red onions, finely sliced
4 tsp honey
2 large handfuls of spinach
  leaves
150g (5oz) goats' cheese
salad, to serve

1. Preheat the grill to high.

2. Crack the eggs into a bowl, add the milk and beat with a fork.

3. Heat the oil in a non-stick frying pan over a medium heat, then add the onions and fry for 8–10 minutes, covered, stirring occasionally, until they soften and brown. Reduce the heat, add the honey and stir well. Fry for a further 1–2 minutes, then add the spinach and stir for 1–2 minutes until it is just starting to wilt.

4. Pour the eggs into the pan and cook for 5-6 minutes until almost set, then break the goats' cheese into chunks and sprinkle them over the top.

5. Place the pan under the hot grill for 3-4 minutes until the egg is set and the cheese is bubbling. Serve with a side salad.

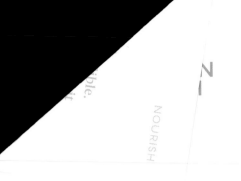
This filling salad is a well-balanced vegetarian meal: the quinoa provides protein, while the rice is full of slow-releasing energy and the avocado is rich in healthy fats. Yum!

SERVES 4

For the salad

400—450g (14oz—1lb) cooked quinoa or wholegrain rice (or a mix of the two)

150g (5oz) sundried tomatoes, drained and chopped

2 large handfuls of spinach, chopped

50g (2oz) flaked almonds

salt and black pepper

For the dressing

1 ripe avocado, halved and stoned

100g (3½oz) natural Greek yoghurt

4 tbsp cold water

4 tbsp chopped coriander

1 large garlic glove

juice of 1 lime

pinch of salt

1. Pop all the salad ingredients in a large bowl, mix together and season to taste.

2. Scoop the flesh of the avocado into a blender, add the remaining dressing ingredients and blitz until smooth and creamy. Pour the dressing over the salad and tuck in!

Tip: Meat eaters can add grilled chicken or fish to this salad for an added protein hit.

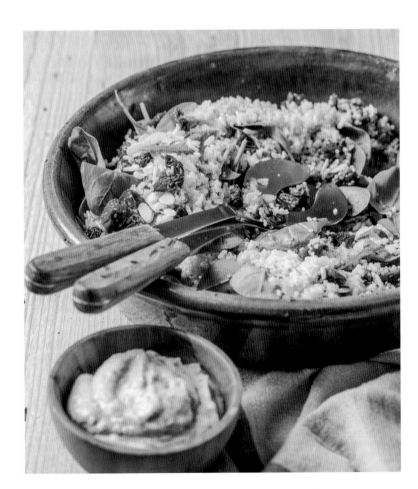

SHAKSHUKA WITH FETA

This is another one you will have seen all over my social media. Shakshuka is just so easy to make that it has become one of my go-to meals. It manages to somehow be both filling and light, and makes a great breakfast or brunch dish, too.

SERVES 2—3

1 tbsp coconut oil

1 red onion, diced

1 large garlic clove, minced

1 large red pepper, seeded and
   roughly chopped

2 x 400g tins of chopped
   tomatoes

2 tbsp tomato puree

½ tsp chilli powder

1 tsp ground cumin

1 tsp paprika

5—6 eggs

1 tbsp chopped flat—leaf
   parsley

120g (4oz) feta

salt and black pepper

1. Heat the oil in a large pan over a medium heat, then add the onion and fry for around 5 minutes until softened and starting to brown. Add the garlic and red pepper and continue cooking for a further couple of minutes until softened, then add the tomatoes, tomato puree and spices and stir well. Simmer over a low-medium heat for 6-7 minutes until the sauce has thickened and reduced. Season to taste.

2. Make 5-6 small wells in the mixture and crack an egg into each well. Pop a lid over the pan and simmer for 5-8 minutes until the eggs are cooked to your liking. Garnish with the chopped parsley and feta and serve warm.

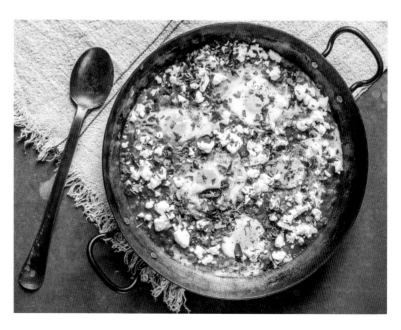

AVOCADO AND VEGGIE RICE PAPER ROLLS WITH DIPPING SAUCE

Vegan friendly!

MAKES 8—10 ROLLS

8—10 rice paper wraps

For the wrap filling

1 Little Gem lettuce, finely
   chopped
50g (2oz) bean sprouts,
   trimmed
1 small carrot, grated
½ cucumber, cut into ribbons
   (unpeeled)
1 medium ripe avocado,
   stoned, peeled and flesh cut
   into strips

For the dipping sauce

3—4 tbsp natural smooth
   almond butter
1 tbsp soy sauce
juice of ½ lime
1 tsp maple syrup
dash of chilli powder (optional)

On my travels around Asia I learnt how to make my own rice paper rolls. I remember thinking that they would make an amazing light lunch or snack, and they most certainly do. Rice paper wraps are a challenge to work with at first, so don't expect your first roll to be a masterpiece. You will soon get the hang of it though!

1. Combine all the sauce ingredients in a bowl, thin the sauce a little with warm water, and set aside.

2. Fill a large heatproof bowl or pan with hot water (not boiling). Place each wrap in the hot water for 10-15 seconds until pliable. Remove and place each wrap on a clean work surface and dab quickly with a clean tea towel to remove excess moisture.

3. Place a selection of the prepared filling ingredients down the centre of one of the wraps (be careful not to overfill it), fold the edge of wrap nearest you over the filling, then fold in the sides and roll up tightly from one end to the other. Repeat with the remaining wraps and filling. Stack them up, dip in, and enjoy.

Tip: You can go wild with the vegetable fillings for these rice paper rolls. Try a combination of any of the following, cut into thin strips: red pepper, radishes, spring onion, raw asparagus, and pack in plenty of fresh herbs such as coriander and mint.

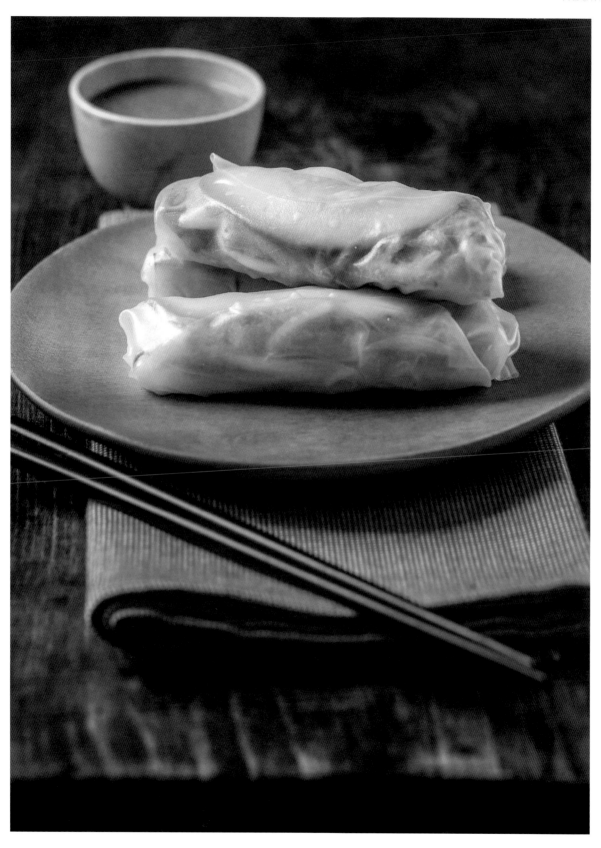

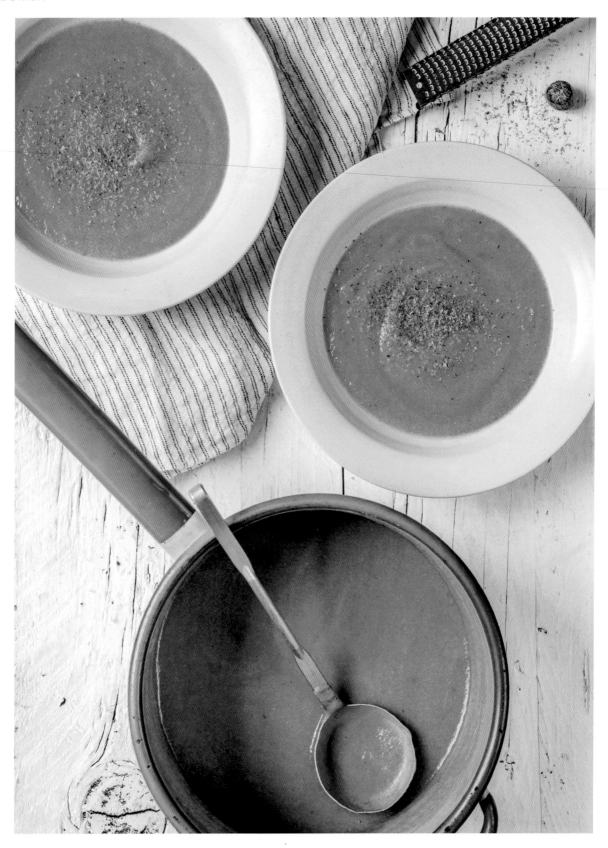

WARMING BUTTERNUT SQUASH SOUP

Vegan friendly!

The cinnamon and nutmeg in this soup rea
cockles in the colder months. Plus, it is pack
micronutrients to keep your immune systen

SERVES 4

1 tbsp coconut oil

1 large onion, chopped

1 red pepper, seeded and
chopped

2 tbsp freshly grated root
ginger

1 garlic clove, minced

1 large butternut squash,
peeled, seeded and chopped

750ml (24fl oz) vegetable stock

½ tsp ground cinnamon

pinch of grated nutmeg

salt and black pepper

1. Heat the oil in a saucepan over a medium heat, then add the onion, red pepper, ginger, garlic and squash and fry for 8 minutes, stirring frequently.

2. Add the stock and bring to the boil, then reduce the heat and simmer for 8-12 minutes, or until squash is tender.

3. Remove from the heat, stir in the cinnamon and season to taste, then blitz with a hand blender until smooth. Serve with a sprinkle of nutmeg on top.

Tip: To inject even more goodness into this soup, add extra red peppers or onions.

CREATE YOUR OWN SALAD

Salads don't have be boring! They can be varied, filling and delicious, and are handy for using up whatever is in your cupboards. This chart shows examples of key ingredients you can combine to build your own personal salad. These are just a few suggestions, the possibilities are endless. Feel free to play around and mix and match. You never know, you might find a new favourite flavour combination!

BASE	CARBS	FATS	PROTEIN	TOPPINGS
Spinach	Roasted sweet potato/squash chunks	Avocado chunks	Chicken	Fresh fruit e.g. pomegranate sees, chopped strawberries, diced apple
Kale	Cooked rice	Nuts	Cooked or smoked fish e.g. salmon	Dried fruit e.g. raisins or chopped apricots
Little Gem lettuce	Cooked quinoa	Cheese — feta or halloumi are my favourites	Cooked shelfish e.g. prawns	Extra veggies e.g. bell pepper or beetroot chunks, grated carrot, chopped radish or tomatoes
Mixed leaves	Cooked couscous	Olives	Cooked red meat	Seeds e.g. pumpkin, sesame or chia
Rocket	Cooked bulgar wheat/other wholegrain	Flaxseeds	Boiled eggs	Fresh herbs e.g. dill or chives

Dressing: Whatever dressing you use, try to keep it light and ideally home-made. My favourite basic dressing is simply 1 teaspoon of white wine vinegar with 1 tablespoon of olive oil whisked together. I then add any additional flavours such as minced garlic, a dash of mustard or some fresh herbs.

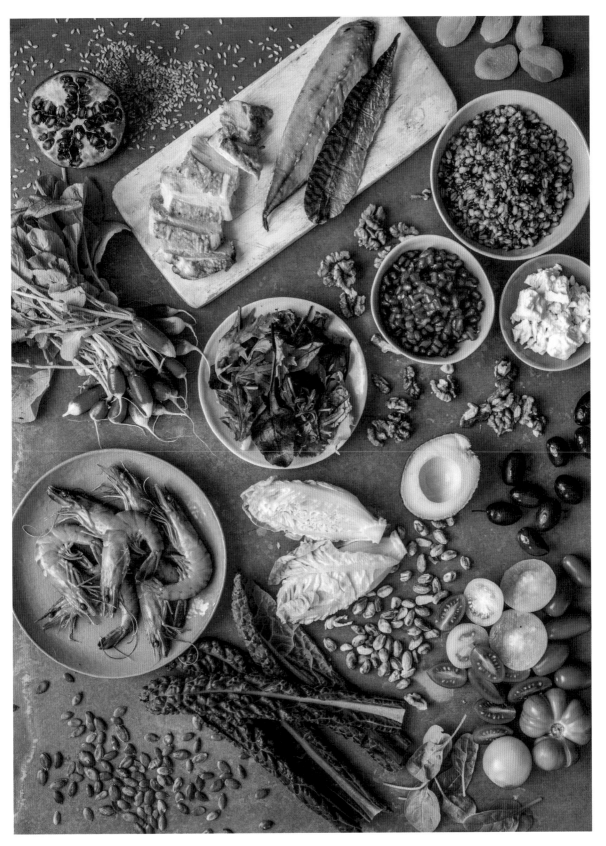

DINNER

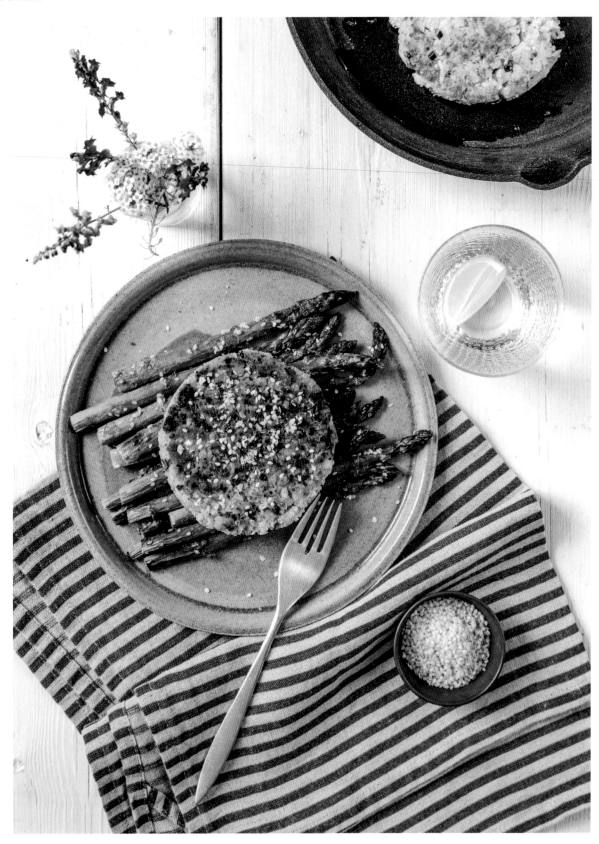

CHICKPEA BURGERS WITH SESAME GARLIC ROASTED ASPARAGUS

Holy moly. This meal is an absolute dream. is filling and flavoursome, and I make the r asparagus all the time as it is just so scrumn

SERVES 4

For the burgers

400g tin of chickpeas, drained, rinsed and patted dry with kitchen paper

grated zest of 1 unwaxed lemon and juice of ½

8 large basil leaves

2 garlic cloves

1 tsp ground cumin

1 egg

100g (3½oz) breadcrumbs

½ red onion, finely diced

coconut oil, for frying

salt and black pepper

For the sesame garlic roasted asparagus

250—300g (9—10oz) asparagus spears

1—2 tbsp olive oil

1 tsp sesame oil

3 large garlic cloves, minced

3 tbsp toasted sesame seeds

pinch of salt

1. Preheat the oven to 220°C/425°F/Gas Mk 7.

2. To make the burgers, simply place all ingredients (except the onions and breadcrumbs) in a food processor and season with salt and pepper. Blitz to form a rough paste. Transfer the burger mixture to a bowl and stir in 75g (2½oz) of the breadcrumbs and all of the diced onion. Form into 4 equal-sized patties and coat the patties in the remaining breadcrumbs. Place on a plate and chill in the fridge for 15 minutes.

3. Meanwhile, toss the asparagus spears in a bowl with the oils, garlic, sesame seeds and salt, then pop them on a baking sheet and bake for 15-20 minutes until tender and crisping up at the tips.

4. When the asparagus is nearly ready, heat some coconut oil in a pan over a medium heat and fry the burgers for 3-5 minutes on each side, until cooked through and golden brown. Remove the asparagus from the oven and serve with the burgers.

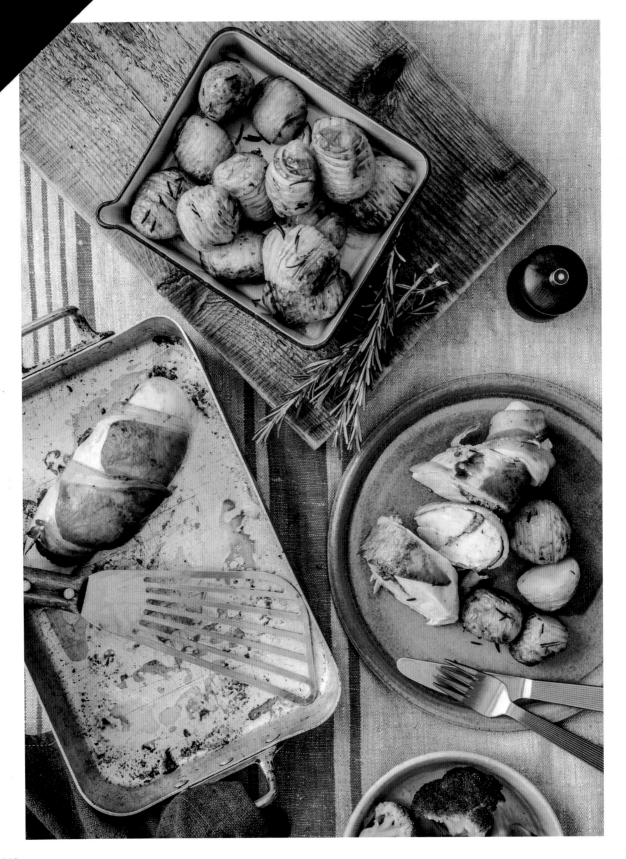

STUFFED CHICKEN WITH HASSELBACK POTATOES

Oh my god. This meal. The potatoes. The chicken. Th[e] bacon. It is so damn good. Trust me!

SERVES 2

For the chicken
2 chicken breasts
4 tsp pesto
2—4 rashers of back bacon

For the hasselback potatoes
500g (1lb 2oz) small new
   potatoes
2 tbsp melted coconut oil
needles from a few sprigs of
   rosemary
salt and black pepper

1. Preheat the oven to 200°C/400°F/Gas Mk 6.

2. First, crack on with the potatoes. Make several incisions along the length of each potato with a sharp knife, 1-2mm apart and going about two thirds of the way through the potato, so that it holds together.

3. Tip the potatoes onto a baking tray, coat them in the melted oil, and sprinkle over the rosemary, pushing some needles into the cuts on each potato. Season with salt and pepper and bake the potatoes for about 50 minutes, turning them halfway through.

4. While the potatoes are roasting, make a deep incision into the side of each chicken breast to create a pocket, being careful not to cut all the way through. Put 2 teaspoons of pesto into each pocket, then wrap 1 or 2 bacon rashers around each breast and secure with a cocktail stick.

5. After the potatoes have been roasting for 30 minutes, transfer the stuffed and wrapped chicken to the roasting tray with the potatoes and roast until the bacon is crisp, the chicken is cooked through, and the potatoes are tender and golden brown.

6. Remove the potatoes and chicken from the oven and serve with vegetables of your choice.

Tip: You can switch the pesto filling for cheese: mozzarella is a classic. If you're feeling super indulgent, sprinkle some coconut sugar on the breasts before you bake them to give them a caramelised crust!

If you follow me on social media you will know that I am a fajita chicken addict! I couldn't not include my signature dinner recipe in this book. You can marinade the chicken in advance, if you like, but it tastes just fine if you don't have time.

SERVES 2 (GENEROUSLY)

2 chicken breasts, finely diced
1 large red onion, finely diced
1 large red pepper, seeded and
　sliced into strips
1 tsp coconut oil
1 ripe avocado
pinch of salt
1 small chilli, finely sliced
　(optional)

For the marinade
1 tbsp smoked paprika
1 tsp ground cumin
½ tsp dried oregano
½ tsp chilli powder
3 tbsp olive oil
2 garlic cloves, crushed
pinch of salt and black pepper

To serve
wholewheat tortillas
cheese of your choice (I like
　feta), grated or crumbled
　(optional)

1. Combine all the marinade ingredients in a bowl. If you're ahead of the game, place the diced chicken in a bowl with three quarters of the marinade, stir to coat, cover and leave to marinate the fridge for a few hours. If not, don't worry: just coat the chicken, onion and pepper in the mixture. If you're marinating the chicken, add the vegetables to the bowl once you're ready to make the fajitas.

2. Heat the coconut oil in a frying pan over a medium heat and add the onion, pepper and chicken coated in the marinade. Fry for about 5 minutes, until the onion and peppers soften and the chicken is nearly cooked through, then add 75ml (3fl oz) water and simmer gently until the water evaporates and everything is softened and cooked through.

3. While the chicken is cooking, halve and stone the avocado, transfer the flesh to a bowl with the salt and mash it to a pulp with the back of a fork.

4. Just before serving, stir the remaining marinade through the chicken to make the meal super-flavourful.

5. Now just stuff the wraps with the chicken and veggie concoction, adding a spoonful of the mashed avocado and anything else you fancy. I personally like a cheeky bit of cheese.

Tip: For a lower carbohydrate meal, substitute the wraps for large lettuce leaves.

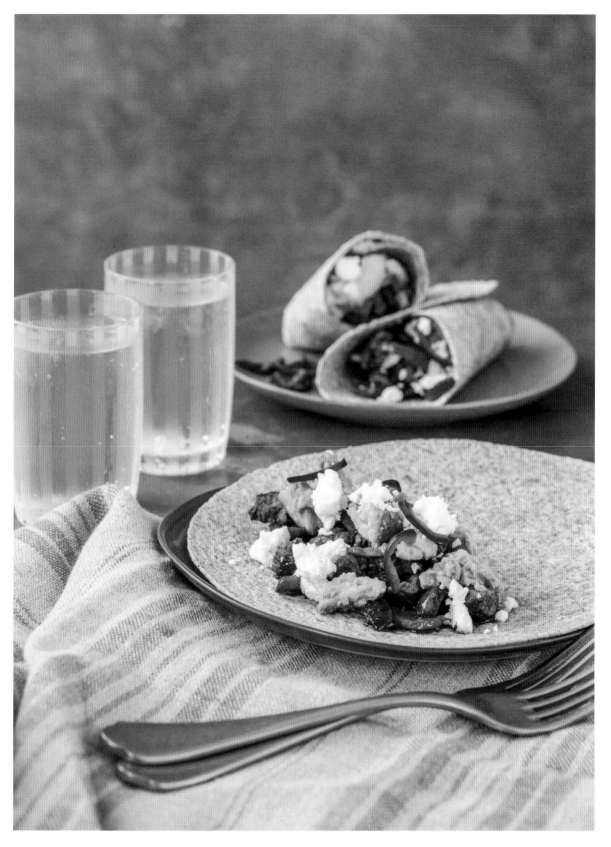

AUBERGINE AND CHICKPEA BAKE

This one-pan wonder is packed full of micronutrients, and can be served as a side dish or as a meal in itself.

SERVES 4—6

1 medium aubergine, cut into
   medium chunks
8 large salad tomatoes, roughly
   chopped
2 courgettes, cut into medium
   chunks
1 red onion, chopped
2 red peppers, seeded and
   chopped
1 tbsp melted coconut oil
1 tbsp dried mixed herbs
6 garlic cloves, peeled and
   roughly chopped
100g (3½oz) roughly chopped
   mushrooms
400g tin of chickpeas, rinsed
   and drained
4 tbsp grated Parmesan
   (optional)
1 tbsp chopped parsley
1 tbsp chopped thyme
grated zest of 1 unwaxed lemon
   and juice of ½ (optional)
salt and black pepper

1. Preheat the oven to 200°C/400°F/Gas Mk 6.

2. Place all the veggies (except the mushrooms and chickpeas) in a roasting tray with the garlic, toss with the oil and dried herbs and roast for 30-40 minutes until brown and tender.

3. Add the mushrooms and chickpeas to the roasting tray (for a cheesy bake, add the Parmesan) and roast for a further 10 minutes, then remove from the oven and stir in the fresh herbs. If you're going for a vegan bake (minus the Parmesan), scatter the bake with the lemon zest and drizzle with the juice.

4. Finally, season to taste and serve.

Tip: This is a meal suitable for all dietary requirements. Meat eaters can serve with it as a side with meat of their choice. Vegetarians can stick with the cheesy option, while vegans can opt for the addition of lemon and scatter the finished dish with toasted nuts for extra crunch (cashews work amazingly!).

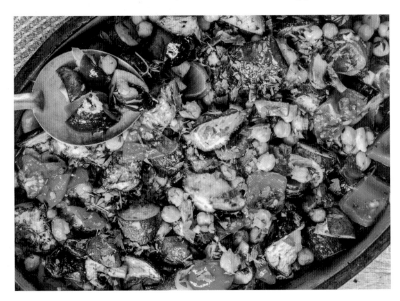

MOROCCAN-SPICED PORK

My mum made this for me all the time when I was younger. It is a Van Dijk family favourite which I am sure you will love, too.

SERVES 3—4

1 tbsp coconut oil
1 large red onion, finely
   chopped
400g (14oz) lean minced pork
2 large garlic cloves, finely
   chopped
1 tbsp medium curry powder
½ tsp ground cumin
2 tbsp tomato puree
400g tin of chopped tomatoes
1 medium red pepper, seeded
   and cut into strips
10 dried apricots, sliced or
   quartered
salt and black pepper
salad or rice, to serve

1. Heat the oil in a heavy-based saucepan over a medium-high heat, add the onions and fry for 3-5 minutes until softened and transparent. Add the pork and fry until brown, breaking the mince up with a wooden spoon as it fries, then add the garlic, curry powder, cumin and tomato puree. Stir to combine and cook for 2 minutes.

2. Add the tinned tomatoes to the pan, then fill the empty tin with water and pour it over. Simmer for 10 minutes, or until most of liquid has evaporated, then tip in the peppers and apricots and cook for a further 5-10 minutes until softened.

3. Season to taste and serve with salad or rice.

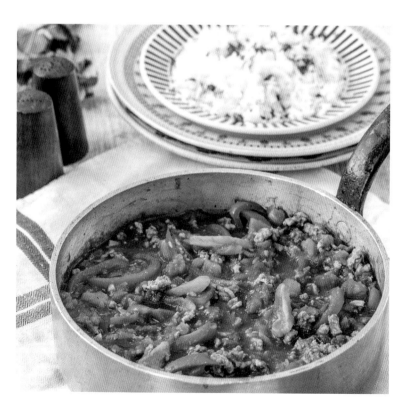

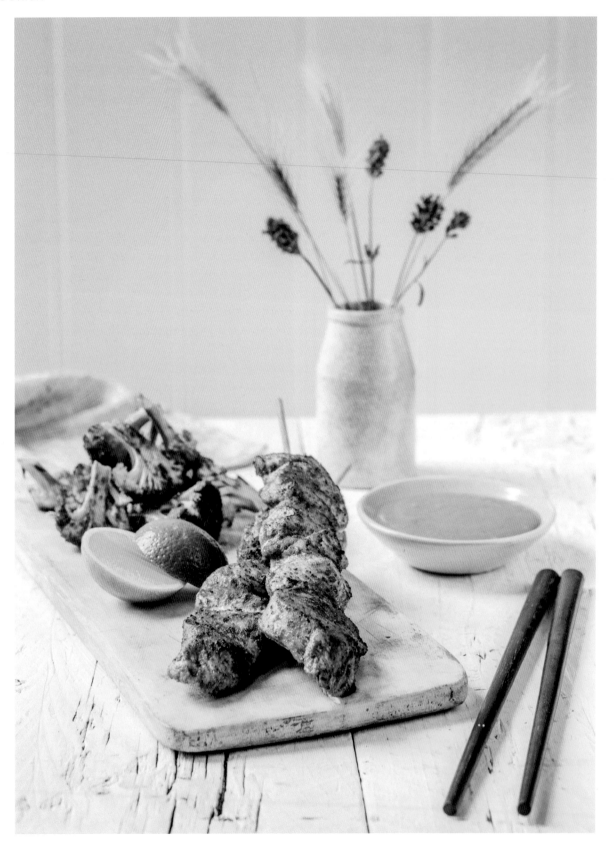

GRILLED SATAY CHICKEN SKEWERS WITH CRISPY BROCCOLI

My obsession with peanut butter has officially crossed from sweet treats into savoury meals. It adds the perfect nutty flavour to this chicken satay dish.

SERVES 2

For the skewers

2 chicken breasts, cut into
  chunky slices
½ tsp salt
½ tsp curry powder (mild,
  medium or hot depending on
  your preference)
1 tbsp melted coconut oil

For the crispy broccoli

1 large head broccoli, cut into
  florets
2 tbsp melted coconut oil
½ tsp salt
pinch of black pepper
grated zest of 1 unwaxed
  lemon
1 large garlic clove, finely diced

For the satay sauce

3 tbsp smooth natural peanut
  butter
3 tbsp full–fat coconut milk
  (from a can — shake the can
  thoroughly before opening)
juice of ½ lime
1 tsp soy sauce
1 tsp clear honey

1. Preheat the oven to 200°C/400°F/Gas Mk 6.

2. Mix the sliced chicken breast in a bowl with the salt, curry powder and coconut oil and transfer to the fridge, covered, to marinate for a minimum of 20 minutes.

3. Toss the broccoli florets in a bowl with the rest of the ingredients, tip onto a greased baking tray and bake in the oven for 15-20 minutes.

4. Thread the marinated chicken strips onto 2 skewers and place on a baking tray. Pop them in the oven with the broccoli and bake for 10 minutes until cooked through, turning halfway through.

5. Meanwhile, make the satay sauce by simply whisking the ingredients together in a bowl.

6. Remove the chicken skewers and broccoli from the oven and serve them immediately, with the sauce in a dish alongside. Bish bash bosh.

THAI SALMON FISHCAKES WITH ROASTED CHERRY TOMATOES

In an ideal world we would all make our own curry paste. The reality is that it can be a bit of a kerfuffle, so if you're short on time don't be afraid to grab a shop-bought one. It's not the end of the world! It makes a great addition to this simple fishcakes recipe.

SERVES 4

4 boneless, skinless salmon
    fillets, cut into chunks
2 tbsp Thai curry paste
1 tbsp freshly grated root
    ginger
1 tsp soy sauce
1 garlic clove, minced
handful of chopped coriander
4 vines of tomatoes
1 tsp melted coconut oil, plus
    extra for frying
salt and black pepper
lime wedges, to serve

1. Preheat the oven to 200°C/400°F/Gas Mk 6.

2. Pop all of the ingredients, except the oil and tomatoes, into a food processor. Pulse until combined into a paste, then use your hands to shape the mixture into 4 patties. Set aside.

3. Place the tomatoes on a roasting tray with a drizzle of the coconut oil and a sprinkling of salt and pepper. Place in the oven for 10 minutes, until the skins start to burst.

4. Meanwhile, heat some coconut oil in a non-stick frying pan over a medium heat and fry the fishcakes for 4-5 minutes on each side until cooked through.

5. Remove the tomatoes from the oven and serve alongside the fishcakes, with lime wedges.

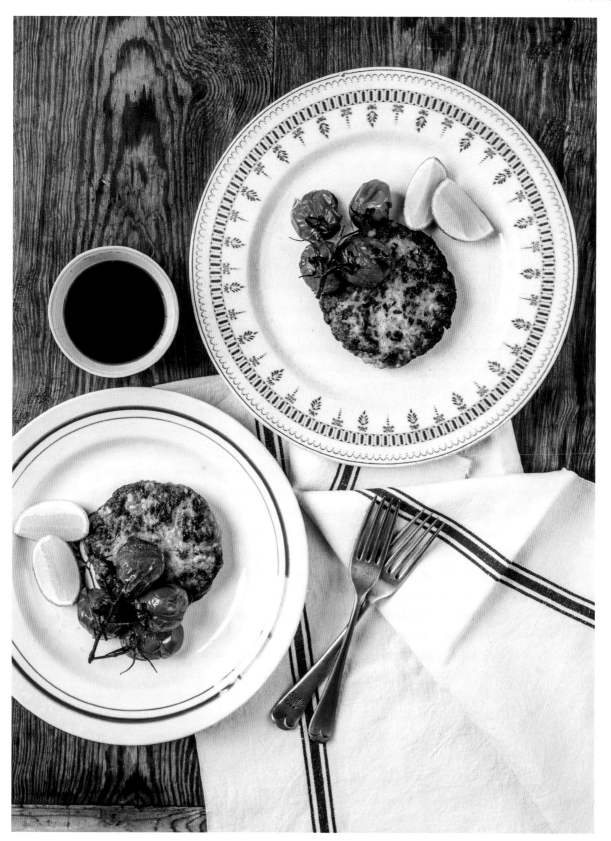

VEGAN 3-BEAN CHILLI
Vegan friendly!

Chilli is the ultimate warming meal in the winter months and this – another one-pot wonder – caters to all dietary requirements. It also stores well in the fridge or freezer so is ideal for making in bulk.

SERVES 4

1 tbsp coconut oil

1 large red onion, diced

3 large garlic cloves, minced

2 red chillies, seeded and diced

2 large celery sticks, very finely chopped

1 large red pepper, seeded and diced

2 x 400g tins of chopped tomatoes

250ml (9fl oz) vegetable stock

4 tbsp tomato puree

400g tin of black beans, drained and rinsed

400g tin of pinto beans, drained and rinsed

400g tin of kidney beans, drained and rinsed

1 tbsp mild chilli powder

2 tsp ground cumin

1 tsp dried oregano

½ tsp smoked paprika

pinch of cayenne pepper (optional)

salt and black pepper

salad or rice, to serve

1. Heat the oil in a frying pan over a medium-high heat, add the onions and garlic and sauté until softened. Add chillies, celery and pepper and sauté for a further 5 minutes, then stir in the chopped tomatoes, stock and tomato puree.

2. Add all the beans, along with the spices (except the cayenne, if using), and simmer for 10-15 minutes until thickened. Taste and if you want it spicier stir in the cayenne and continue to cook for a further 1-2 minutes.

3. Remove from the heat, season to taste, and serve with salad or some rice.

Tip: If you're a meat eater, feel free to add lean minced meat after sautéing the onions.

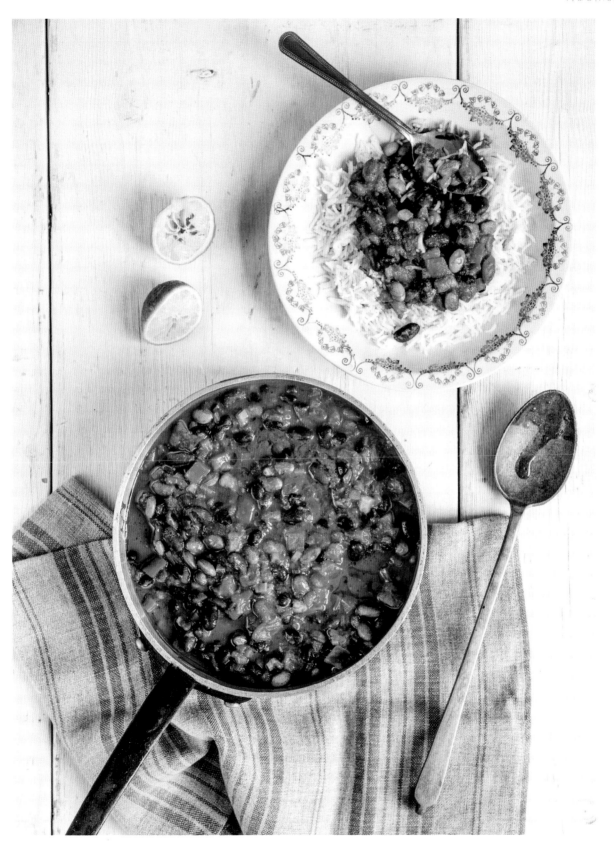

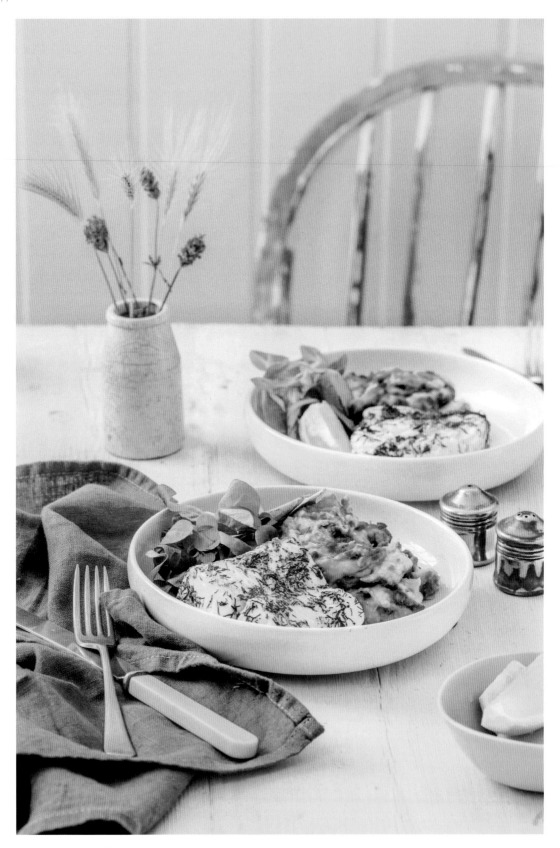

LEMON AND DILL POLLOCK WITH SWEET POTATO AND BEETROOT MASH

Pollock is a cheap and widely available fish that you can easily jazz up with the delicious flavours of lemon and dill.

SERVES 2

2 skinless pollock fillets
  (or fillets from another firm,
  white sustainable fish)
4 tbsp finely chopped dill
4 tbsp freshly squeezed lemon
  juice
1 tbsp melted coconut oil
½ tbsp Dijon mustard
1 garlic clove, minced
pinch of salt
pinch of black pepper
cooking spray

**For the sweet potato
and beetroot mash**
500g (1lb 2oz) sweet potatoes,
  peeled and cut into chunks
2 cooked beetroots (not in
  vinegar), cut into chunks
2 tbsp natural Greek yoghurt
salt and black pepper

1. Place the pollock fillets in a bowl or plastic food bag, add the dill, lemon juice, coconut oil, mustard and garlic, season with salt and pepper, mix gently, cover the bowl or seal the bag and leave to marinate in the fridge for around 20 minutes. Preheat the oven to 200°C/400°F/Gas Mk 6.

2. Meanwhile, bring a pan of salted water to the boil, add the sweet potato chunks, reduce the heat and simmer for 10 minutes until tender. Add the beetroot and simmer for a further 2 minutes, then drain, transfer to a bowl, add the yoghurt and mash all together, adding salt and pepper to taste. Keep warm while you cook the fish.

3. Once the fish has marinated, wrap the fillets individually in foil, place on a baking tray and bake in the oven for 15 minutes, or until cooked through.

4. Remove the fish from the oven, unwrap the foil and serve with the sweet potato and beetroot mash.

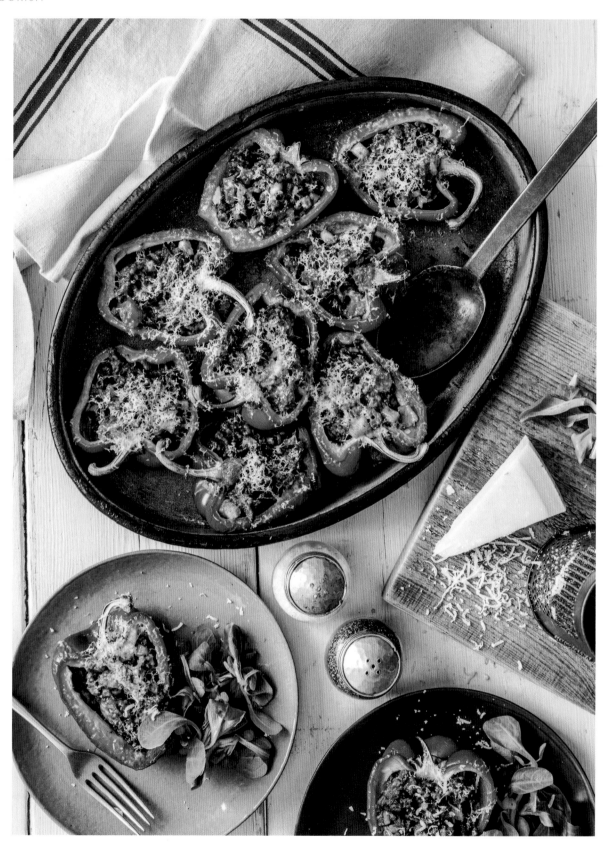

SPICY BEEF STUFFED PEPPERS

Here's another Van Dijk family favourite for you. is a farmer and we frequently have an abundance peppers which need eating, and are always findin things to stuff them with. This is my favourite!

SERVES 6

6 large red peppers, halved and
  seeded (leave the stalks on)
coconut oil, melted, for frying
1 large red onion, diced
500g (1lb 2oz) lean beef mince
2 garlic cloves, crushed
1 large courgette, finely diced
100g (3½oz) mushrooms,
  finely diced
1 red chilli, seeded and chopped
1 beef stock cube
2 x 400g tins chopped
  tomatoes
4 tbsp tomato puree
1 tbsp dried mixed herbs
100g (3½oz) grated Parmesan
salt and black pepper

1. Preheat the oven to 200°C/400°F/Gas Mk 6.

2. Place the peppers on a baking tray cut side up and drizzle with a tablespoon of melted coconut oil. Roast for 15–20 minutes until they are beginning to soften, then remove and place cut side up in a baking dish. Leave the oven on.

3. Heat 1 teaspoon of coconut oil in a heavy-based saucepan over a medium-high heat, add the onion and cook until softened, then add the mince and fry, breaking up the mince with a wooden spoon, until browned. Add the garlic, courgette, mushrooms and chilli and cook for 2–3 minutes, then crumble in the stock cube, tip in the tinned tomatoes, add the tomato puree and the mixed herbs. Bring to the boil, reduce the heat and simmer for 15 minutes, stirring frequently, until the vegetables are tender and the liquid has reduced. Season to taste.

4. Divide the sauce between the pepper cavities, sprinkle with the Parmesan and bake for 10–15 minutes, until the cheese is crispy and the sauce is bubbling. Remove from the oven and serve warm with side dishes of your choice.

Tip: You will probably be left with some mince filling that won't fit in the peppers. Store it in a container and eat the next day with salad (although my favourite way of using up the leftovers is to have it on toast!).

THE SWEET STUFF

LEMON CHIA ENERGY BALLS
Vegan friendly!

MAKES 5—6 BALLS

15 large pitted dates
35g (1¼oz) walnuts
2 tbsp unsweetened
    desiccated coconut
2 tbsp chia seeds
grated zest of 1
    unwaxed lemon

These zesty energy balls take just minutes to make, can be made in advance, and are the perfect, energising on-the-go snack.

1. Just chuck all the ingredients in a food processor and blitz until they form a thick paste.

2. Use your hands to mould the mixture into 5-6 equal-sized balls.

3. Store in an airtight container in the fridge for up to 5 days.

Tip: Switch the walnuts for any nut of your choice: almonds are particularly good in this recipe.

BOUNTY PROTEIN BALLS

MAKES 6—8 BALLS

3 scoops (75g/2½oz) chocolate
    protein powder
25g (1oz) cocoa powder
1 tbsp clear honey
40g (1½oz) porridge oats
40g (1½oz) unsweetened
    desiccated coconut, plus
    extra for rolling
75ml (3fl oz) milk
pinch of salt

These protein balls are an easy-to-make, portable and high protein snack packed with natural energy.

1. Combine all the ingredients in a bowl to form a thick paste.

2. Use your hands to mould the batter into 6–8 equal-sized balls, then roll them in extra desiccated coconut.

3. Store in an airtight container in the fridge for up to 5 days.

Tip: Depending on the protein powder you use, the batter can end up a smidge too wet or too dry. If it's too wet, add extra protein powder or cocoa powder; If it's too dry add a dash of milk.

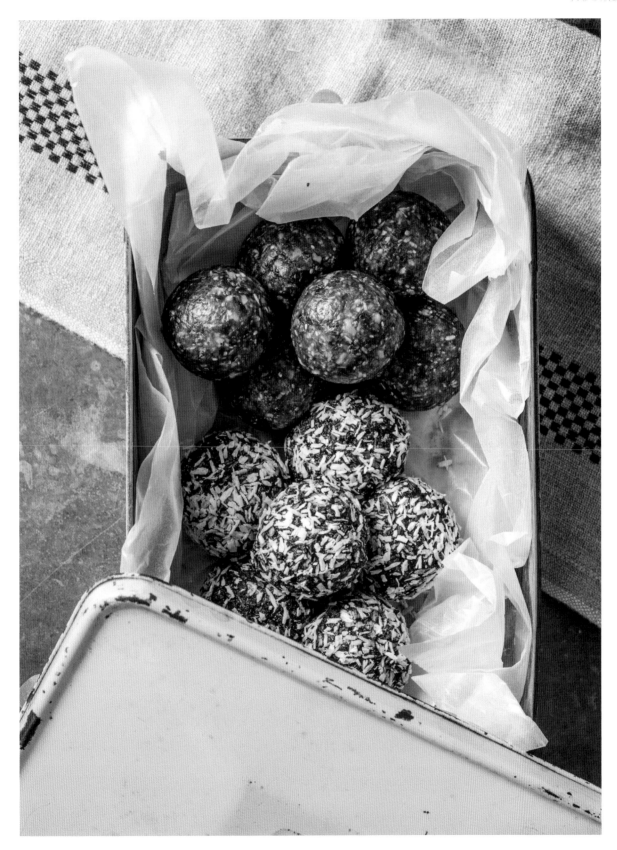

WARM AND GOOEY STUFFED DATES
Vegan friendly!

SERVES 2

4 large medjool dates, pitted
4 tsp natural nut butter (I
   love smooth cashew butter or
   crunchy almond butter)
dark chocolate chips or
   chopped nuts, to serve

These dates are a delicious and indulgent sweet treat, packed with natural energy and healthy fats to keep you feeling satiated.

1. Preheat the oven to 180°C/350°F/Gas Mk 4.

2. Stuff each date with a teaspoonful of nut butter. Pop the dates on a baking tray and bake in the oven for 2-3 minutes, until warm and gooey.

3. Remove from the oven, add any toppings you like and eat while they're still warm. Divine!

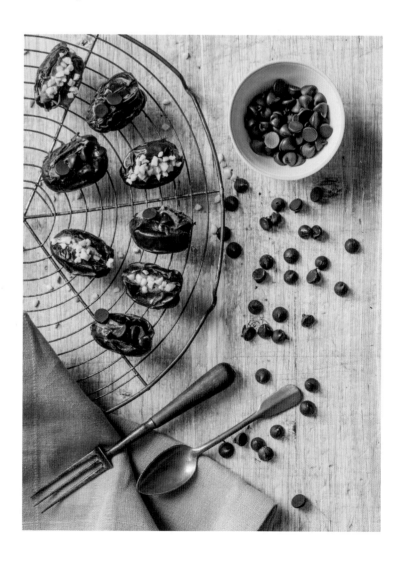

THE ULTIMATE HEALTHY COOKIES

Seriously guys, these cookies are the badger's nadgers. The bee's knees. The dog's hoo-haa's. It will take every ounce of your self control not to eat the whole batch!

MAKES 6 COOKIES

150g (5oz) ground almonds
2 tbsp clear honey
1 tsp vanilla extract
¼ tsp baking powder
3 tbsp coconut oil or good quality grass–fed butter, melted
2 tbsp dark chocolate chips or chopped dark chocolate (70% cocoa solids)

1. Preheat the oven to 180°C/350°F/Gas Mk 4 and line a large baking sheet with baking parchment.

2. Combine all the ingredients in a bowl, then use your hands to form 6 balls of mixture and place them on the baking sheet, pressing them down with your hands until they are roughly 7cm diameter and 1cm thick.

3. Bake the cookies for 8-10 minutes, until golden brown and set at the edges but soft in the middle. Remove from the oven and leave them to cool and set on the baking sheet.

Tip: Not a chocolate fan? (You're mad!) Then you can substitute the chocolate chips with raisins or dried cranberries.

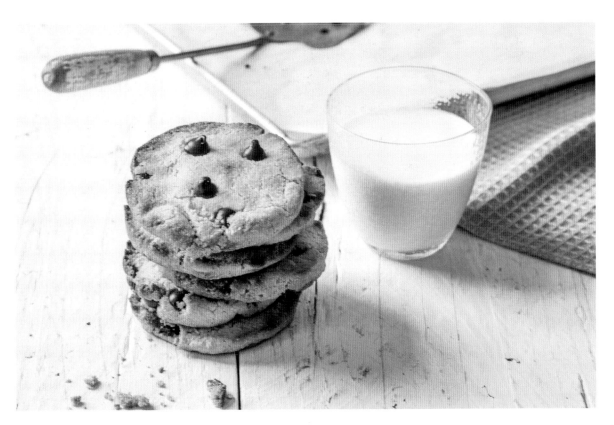

THE ULTIMATE BROWNIES

These brownies are so fudgy, gooey and delicious; you would never suspect that they are healthy or that they contain a sneaky bit of veg!

MAKES 10–12 BROWNIES

115g (3⅔oz) porridge oats
2 small cooked beetroots
    (about 100g/3½oz), drained
    and puréed (you can use
    ready-cooked beetroot, but
    not in vinegar)
3 medium eggs, lightly beaten
50g (2oz) cocoa powder, sifted
    if lumpy
150g (5oz) clear honey
4 tbsp melted coconut oil
1 tsp baking powder
1 tsp vanilla extract

1. Preheat the oven to 170°C/325°F/Gas Mk 3 and line a 22cm square baking tin (minimum 2.5cm deep) with baking parchment.

2. Blitz the oats in a blender or food processor until a fine flour is formed. Tip into a mixing bowl.

3. Place the cooked and drained beetroot in the blender or food processor and blitz to form a puree, then add the puree to the oats.

4. Combine the oat flour and the beetroot puree with the remaining ingredients and pour into the lined tray. Bake for 12 minutes on the middle shelf of the oven, or until cooked through but still slightly soft in the middle.

5. Remove from the oven and leave to cool in the tin before slicing.

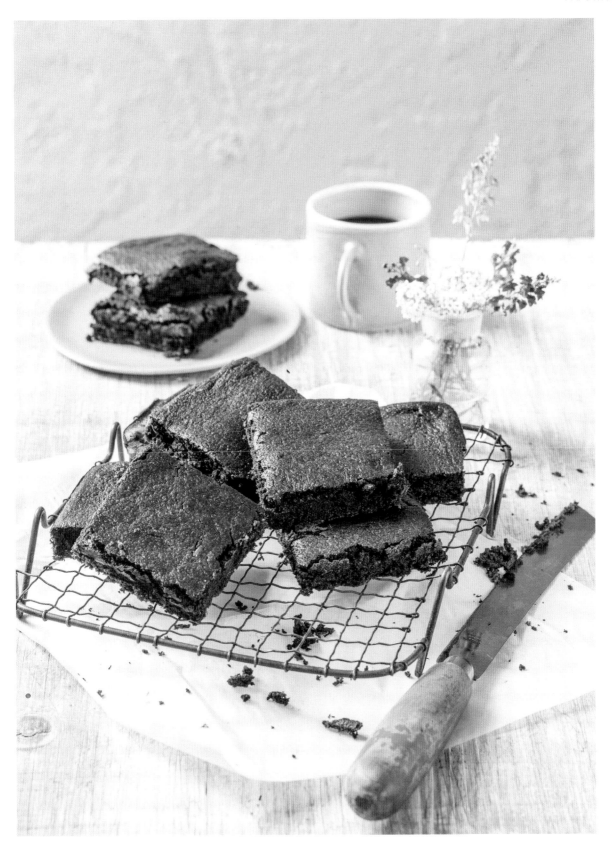

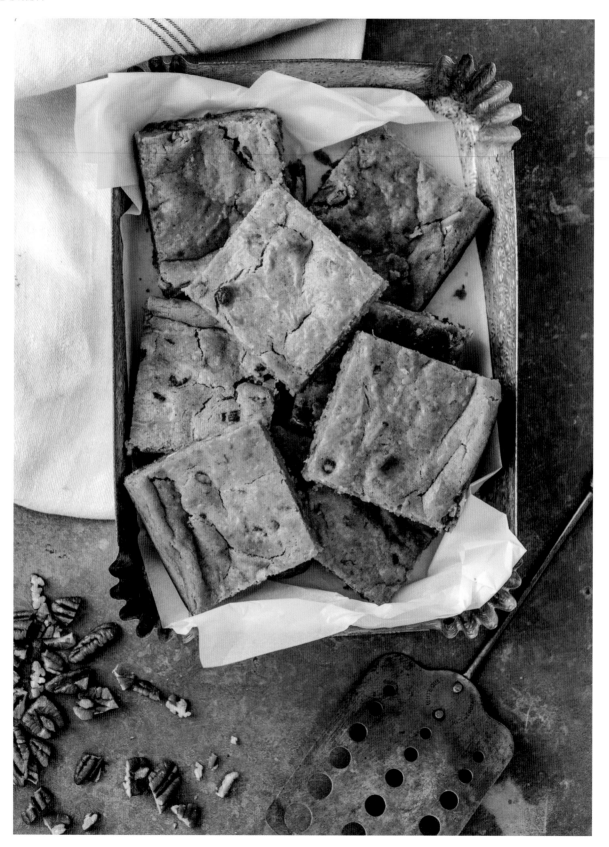

WHITE CHOCOLATE PECAN BLONDIES

Yep, these blondies contain chickpeas. Sounds bizarre. Tastes amazing. I swear these are so indulgent, even your grandma would approve!

MAKES 12 BLONDIES

400g tin of chickpeas, drained and rinsed
180ml (6fl oz) milk
85g (2¾oz) clear honey
1 tsp baking powder
1 tsp vanilla extract
250g (9oz) natural smooth peanut butter
50g (2oz) roughly chopped pecans
50g (2oz) white chocolate chips or chopped white chocolate

1. Preheat the oven to 180°C/350°F/Gas Mk 4 and line a 20 x 30cm tray (minimum 2.5cm deep) with baking parchment.

2. Blitz the chickpeas in a blender or food processor with the milk to form a smooth batter.

3. Transfer the batter to a bowl and add the honey, baking powder, vanilla extract and peanut butter. Stir in the pecans and chocolate chips and transfer the mixture to the lined baking tray. Bake for 20-25 minutes, until cooked through and golden brown at the edges, but still a little soft in the middle.

4. Remove from the oven and leave to cool and set in the tin. This can take a while, so I often pop them in the fridge for 1 hour, once they've reached room temperature. Once set, cut into 12 slices or squares and enjoy!

Tip: These blondies may contain more natural wholesome ingredients, but they are still indulgent and should be treated as such. I know it can be hard, since they taste like the elixir of life, but try to consume them in moderation.

BANANA POPS

These banana pops are the perfect snack for warm summer days, and are a fun treat to make with children.

MAKES 4 POPS

2 large bananas, peeled and
  halved widthways
150g (5oz) dark chocolate
  (minimum 70% cocoa solids),
  chopped

Toppings
unsweetened desiccated coconut
chopped nuts
chocolate chips

1. Pop each banana half on the end of a lolly stick, and line a baking tray with foil.

2. Melt the chocolate in a heatproof bowl over a pan of simmering water (making sure the bottom of the bowl doesn't touch the water), or in the microwave on High in 30-second bursts.

3. Fully immerse the bananas in the melted chocolate, turning them to make sure they're completely covered, then place them on the foil-lined tray. Sprinkle over toppings of your choice, then transfer to the freezer for at least 1 hour before serving.

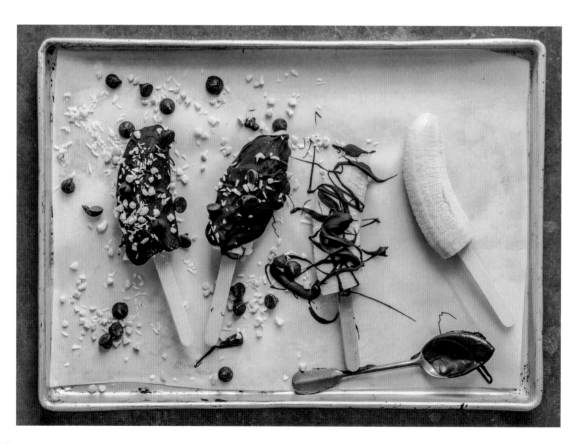

BANANA PEANUT BUTTER ICE CREAM

Both sweet and nutty, this ice cream takes just 2 minutes to make and makes for a more natural dessert or summer snack. The quantities below make one serving, but can easily be increased to serve more people.

SERVES 1

2 medium peeled bananas, frozen

1 heaped tbsp peanut butter

3 tbsp milk

1. Pop the ingredients in a blender or food processor and blitz until smooth. You might need to remove the blender lid and stir the ingredients once or twice to help them combine.

2. Serve immediately for a soft-serve texture (my favourite!), or freeze to achieve a traditional ice cream consistency.

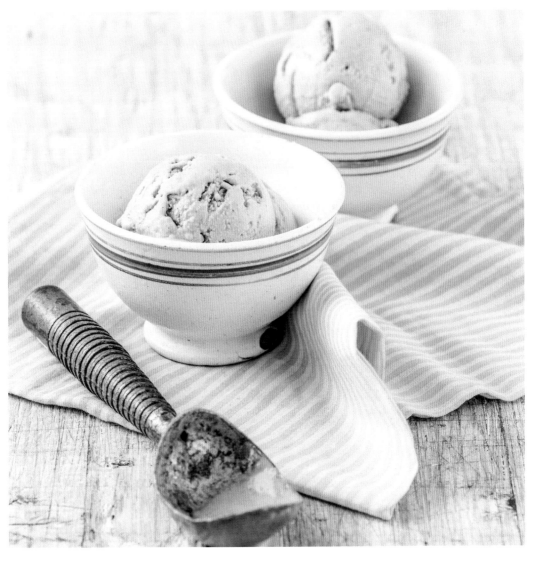

SINGLE SERVING PROTEIN BROWNIE

What if I told you that you can make a delicious gooey brownie, which contains 20g of protein, in a matter of minutes? Prepare to have your mind blown.

MAKES 1 BROWNIE

1 scoop (20g/¾oz)
   chocolate whey protein
   powder
10g (⅓oz) cocoa powder
½ tsp baking powder
about 3 tbsp milk

1. Pop all the ingredients in a microwaveable mug. Stir to combine until a stiff batter is formed.

2. Microwave on High for 30 seconds for a molten centre, or 45 seconds–1 minute for a fully fledged brownie.

3. Serve as you like. I tend to have mine with yoghurt and fruit.

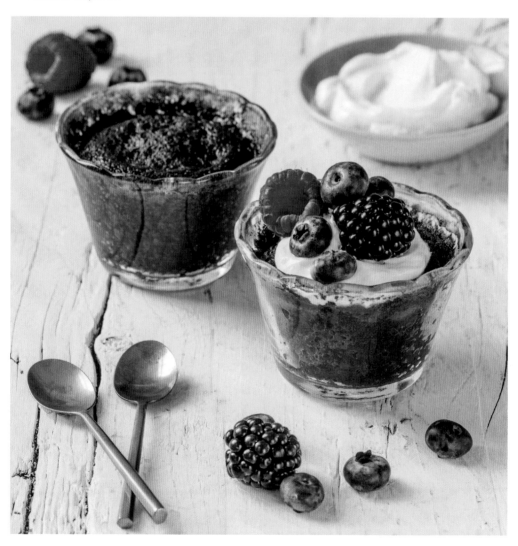

PUMPKIN SPICE BAKED APPLES

A true people pleaser; this warming treat can be made any time of year but is particularly delicious in the autumn.

SERVES 4

coconut oil, for greasing
4 large cooking apples
100g (3½oz) porridge oats
1 tsp ground cinnamon
35g (1¼oz) chopped dates
30g (1oz) chopped pecans
1 tbsp maple syrup
1 tsp vanilla extract
100ml (3½fl oz) milk

1. Preheat the oven to 170°C/325°F/Gas Mk 3 and grease and line a baking dish.

2. Wash and core the apples, making a hole in the centre about 2.5cm (1in) wide, for maximum stuffing capacity. Pop the apples in the lined dish.

3. Combine the remaining ingredients in a bowl and fill the apples with the batter, ensuring it fills the entire cavity, all the way through the core. If there is any leftover mixture just sprinkle it on the tray and it will make a yummy crunchy topping.

4. Bake for 30-50 minutes (the cooking time will depend on which variety of apple you're using), until cooked through and a fork can be easily inserted into an apple. Remove from the oven and serve warm, with the extra mixture scattered on top, if you have any. I love mine with yoghurt and even more cinnamon sprinkled on top.

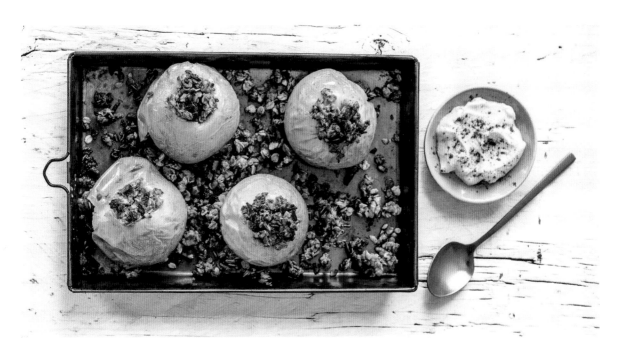

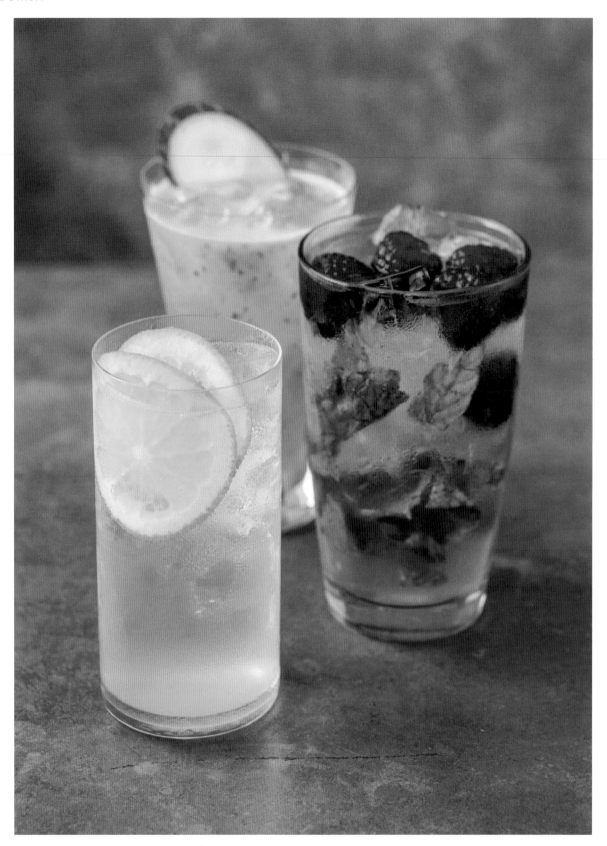

CUCUMBER AND ELDERFLOWER COOLER

You can omit the honey from this zingy cocktail for a sharper flavour, or add it in to keep things sweet!

SERVES 1

⅓ large cucumber
2 tbsp elderflower cordial
1 measure vodka
handful of ice cubes
soda water

1. Place the cucumber in a blender or food processor and blitz to form a puree.

2. Pour the cucumber puree into a large glass and add the elderflower cordial and vodka. Mix until combined, then add the ice and top up with soda water.

ORANGE GIN AND TONIC

This fruity twist on a classic gin and tonic is refreshing and zesty.

SERVES 1

juice of ½ large orange
1 measure gin
1 tbsp clear honey (optional)
2 orange slices
handful of ice cubes
tonic water

1. Mix the orange juice, gin and honey together (if using) in a large glass.

2. Add the orange slices and ice to the glass, then top up the glass with tonic water.

RASPBERRY AND MINT MOJITO

Combining fruity and fresh flavours, this mojito is light and delicious.

SERVES 1

juice of ½ lime
12 mint leaves
1 tbsp clear honey
1 measure white rum
5 fresh raspberries
handful of ice cubes
soda water

1. Roughly mix together the lime juice, mint leaves and honey in a large glass to release the flavour from the leaves. Set aside for 1 minute.

2. Add the rum and raspberries to the glass. Fill the glass with ice and top up with soda water.

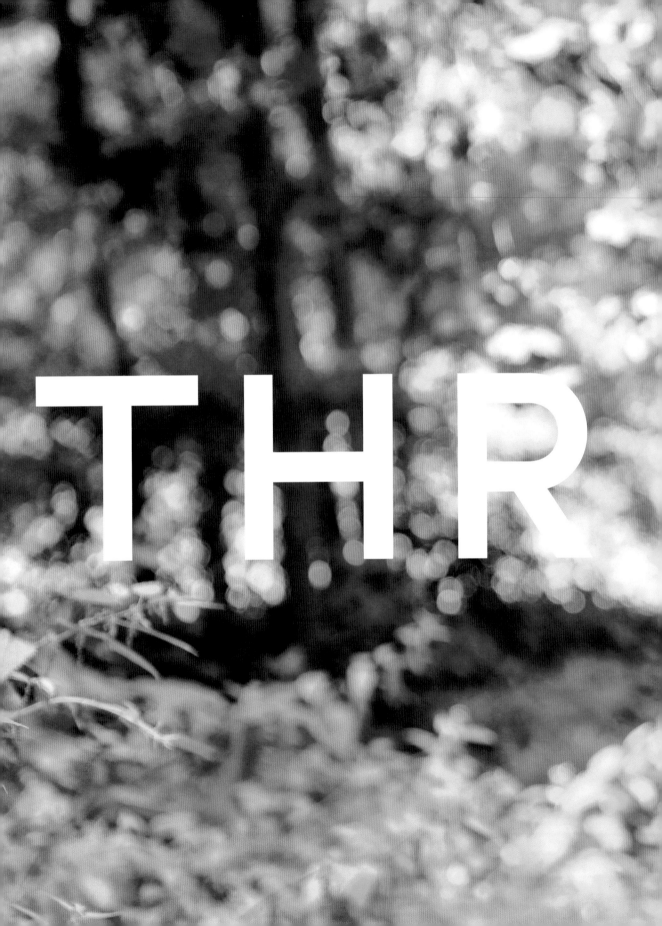

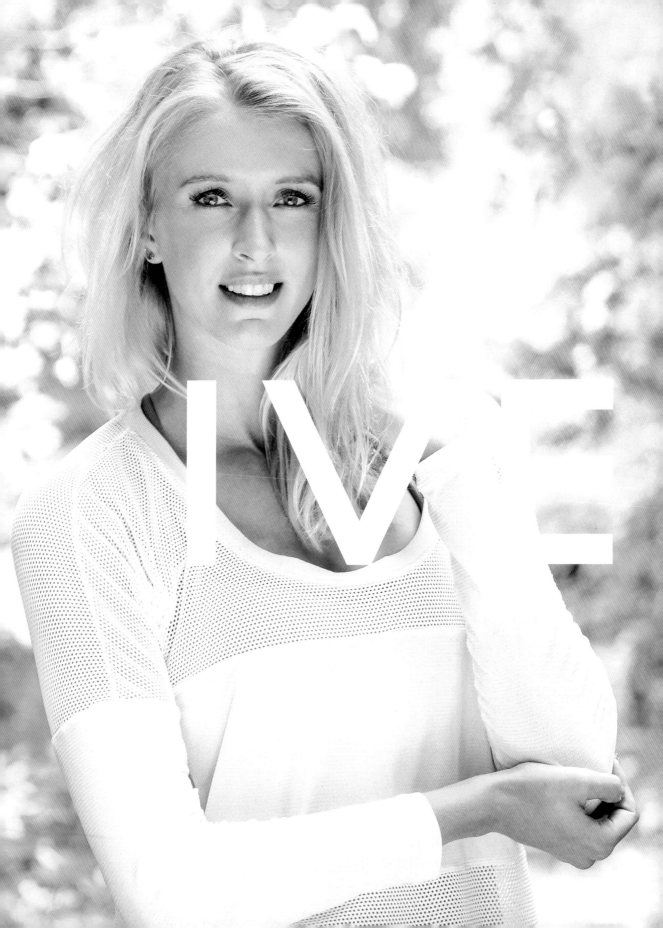

IT'S YOUR TIME TO THRIVE

So that's it – that is all of my tips, tricks and secrets which you can apply to your life to achieve lasting results. It's time to start implementing some positive changes. Here are my simple steps to get you started on your road to becoming fitter, healthier and happier.

The first thing I recommend doing is reflecting. Really take some time to reflect on where you are now with your training and nutrition, your body image and your happiness. Write down how you feel if you like, as this can help you to more clearly organise your thoughts. As part of this reflection and self-evaluation, I always recommend making a food diary for a week or tracking your food using an app such as MyFitnessPal. This allows you to notice anything you're over- or under-eating and gives you a valuable insight into your dietary intake.

The second step is to look internally and ask yourself what your goals are, what motivates you and what will truly make you happy. Be honest with yourself and don't try and think the 'right thing', just allow yourself to be made aware of what you **really** want to do and achieve. No judgement. Use this knowledge to set yourself realistic goals with regard to both your health and your life. It is really rewarding to write these things down and come back to reflect on them in the future. It can be amazing to see how far you have come.

The third step is to make changes to your lifestyle. There are two ways you can do this. The first is to go cold turkey and to completely and utterly overhaul your life. This works for some but not all; however, if you prefer this approach then fair play – go smash it. The second approach, and the one I personally advocate, is to use a process of modification. This involves identifying small, achievable and sustainable modifications you can make to your existing lifestyle. This could be anything from having a balanced breakfast to drinking two litres of water a day or adding in an extra workout a week. Once you have mastered these, you can start adding in more modifications until eventually you've achieved the healthy lifestyle you set out to implement. Ultimately what matters is that you find an approach that works for **you**.

FINDING YOUR BALANCE

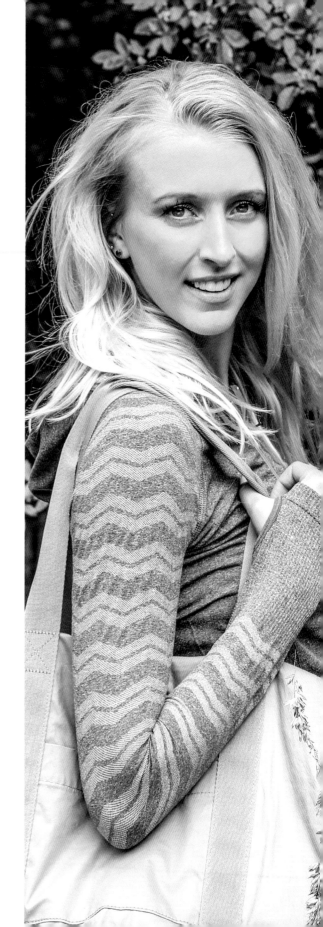

Embarking on a healthier lifestyle is a new and exciting challenge and one I am certain you're ready to face. On this journey remember why you're making these changes and know that what you're doing right now is affecting the health and happiness of your current and future self. What you put into your body affects you in so many ways beyond how you look. Nourish your body with wholesome foods. Move it in ways you enjoy. Develop a healthy mindset. Look after yourself and let yourself become the person you want to be. Live your life to the fullest. By picking up this book you've already moved one step ahead of everyone else, so keep on going.

I hope that *Strong* has opened your eyes to how enjoyable and achievable living a healthy lifestyle can be. I have given you the tools to make lasting and positive changes to your life, and hopefully I have set you on a path to become the fittest, healthiest and happiest version of you. Reading this book is only the start of your journey. Keep learning. Implement positive changes. Change your life for the better. Stay consistent and do it for the right reasons. Enjoy the journey.

You've got this. Zanna xx

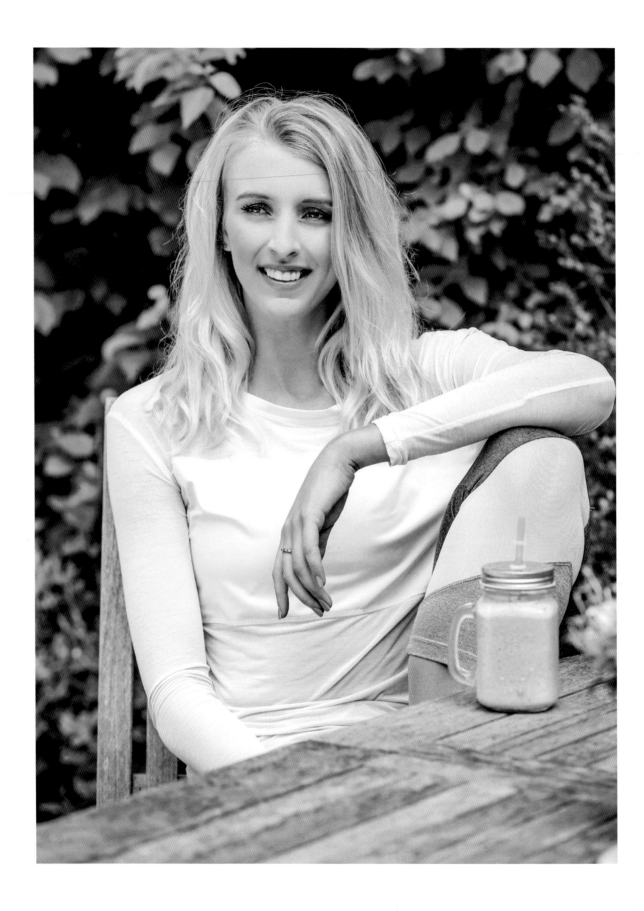

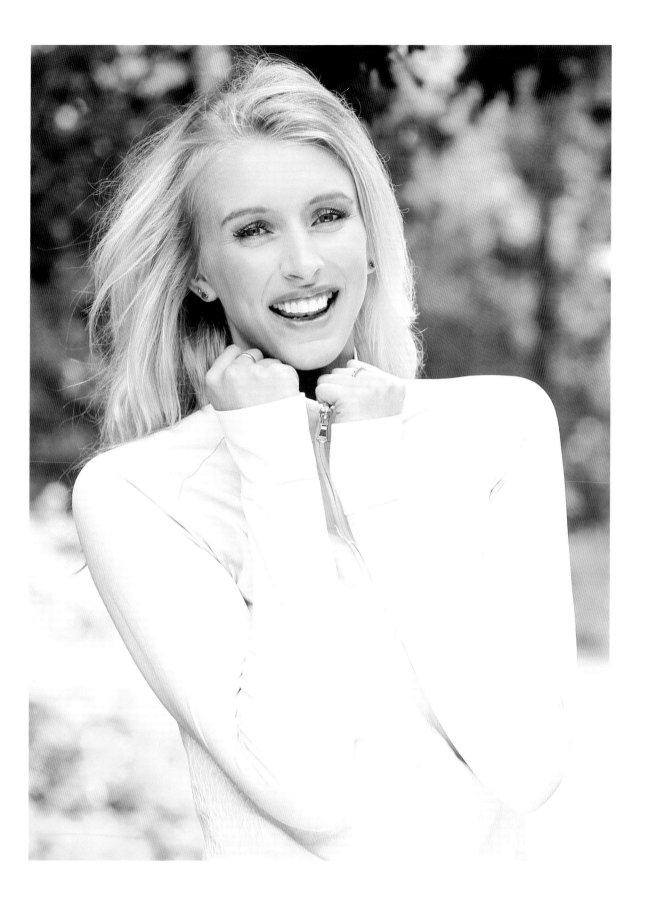

INDEX

RECIPE INDEX